Praise for the *Make Your Brain Smarter* Approach

"Chapman's broader idea—that smarts come with consistent practice—and her pragmatic 'brain health plan' are intriguing."

—*Publishers Weekly*

"Chapman's program encourages thinking broadly and creatively to stimulate the frontal lobe. Considering that she created a program designed to sharpen the minds of Navy SEALs in the same way their elite training hones their bodies, you may want to toss the crosswords and give this a try."

—*BookPage*

"I don't want to grow old and feel bad, either physically or mentally. That's why I exercise my body and my brain daily. I'm well into my eighties. I know that half my life is over, and that keeping my brain challenged is more important than ever. Thanks to the pioneering brain research being done by Dr. Sandi Chapman, we can have healthy and productive minds for far longer than we might have imagined."

—T. Boone Pickens, legendary entrepreneur, innovator,
energy executive, and author of *The First Billion Is the Hardest:
Reflections on a Life of Comebacks and America's Energy Future*

"As someone who strives to learn more, communicate more effectively, and be more productive, and to strengthen my strategic thinking and creative innovation every single day, I wholeheartedly live by Sandi Chapman's guide to making our brain smarter. The topic of brain health is critical to our future as we all want to continue to live strong, vibrant, impactful lives for as long as we possibly can."

—Melissa Reiff, president of The Container Store

"As an athlete, I always knew the importance of training my body for optimal performance. It wasn't until I met Sandi Chapman that I learned that the same is true for my brain. It has eased my concerns about my future health after spending more than ten years in the impact lifestyle of the NFL."

—Daryl Johnston, former Dallas Cowboy,
NFL commentator, and business leader

"The BrainHealth physical and the SMART program let me know how I could reach my full cognitive potential. These strategies revolutionized my life and could change the lives of millions. In the knowledge era, cognitive performance has never been more needed, but the distractions are great and growing. This book comes at the perfect time."

— Donovan Campbell, *New York Times* bestselling author
of *Joker One* and *The Leader's Code*

"SMART training truly changed my life. I can't think of any other training I've had that has delivered benefits so quickly and deeply."

—Laura Sanford, regional vice president, AT&T

"I've had annual physicals for more than thirty years, so it made sense to check the top third of the body also. Taking the BrainHealth Physical gave me a sense of peace knowing that I had a baseline of my brain function and could measure any issues that arise in the future."

—Lyda Hill, a philanthropreneur

"When I learned of the research of Dr. Sandi Chapman, I immediately realized her work could be transformational in accelerating the brain performance of employees at all ages. As the global leader of human resources, I am always looking for ways to expand the diverse talents of the different generational age groups that all too often go underdeveloped. Both companies and the individuals will be the beneficiaries of better brain health."

—Cynthia Brinkley, Vice President of
Global Human Resources, General Motors

"The profoundly effective program outlined in *Make Your Brain Smarter* uses relatively simple and straightforward strategies to empower learners. The program allowed my son to believe in himself, created a level playing field for him to pursue his dreams, and utilized his talents without barrier deficits. We have seen a dramatic improvement in his brain performance, and I know the strategies will continue to have a positive impact on his life and continued success for years to come."

—David Waldrep, entrepreneur and father whose son
participated in teen high-performance brain training

MAKE YOUR BRAIN
SMARTER

Increase Your Brain's Creativity,
Energy, and Focus

SANDRA BOND CHAPMAN, Ph.D.
with Shelly Kirkland

Simon & Schuster Paperbacks
New York   London   Toronto   Sydney   New Delhi

Simon & Schuster Paperbacks
A Division of Simon & Schuster, Inc.
1230 Avenue of the Americas
New York, NY 10020

First Simon & Schuster trade paperback edition January 2014

SIMON & SCHUSTER PAPERBACKS and colophon are trademarks of Simon & Schuster, Inc.

For information about special discounts for bulk purchases, please contact Simon & Schuster Special Sales at 1-866-506-1949 or *business@simonandschuster.com*.

The Simon & Schuster Speakers Bureau can bring authors to your live event. For more information or to book an event contact the Simon & Schuster Speakers Bureau at 1-866-248-3049 or visit our website at *www.simonspeakers.com*.

Designed by Carla Jayne Jones

Manufactured in the United States of America

10   9   8   7   6   5   4   3   2

The Library of Congress has cataloged the hardcover edition as follows:
Chapman, Sandra Bond.
  Make your brain smarter : increase your brain's creativity, energy, and focus / Sandra Bond Chapman with Shelly Kirkland.—1st ed.
    p. cm.
  Includes bibliographical references and index.
  Thought and thinking. 2. Cognition. 3. Brain. 4. Neurosciences. I. Kirkland, Shelly. II. Title.
  BF441.C3633 2013
  153—dc23   2012024798

ISBN 978-1-4516-6547-5
ISBN 978-1-4516-6548-2 (pbk)
ISBN 978-1-4516-6549-9 (ebook)

Chart on page 172: Used with permission, MetLife Mature Market Institute 2012. All rights reserved.

To Don: one of the smartest and most compassionate men ever

To Noah: for showing me the evolution of smart in the younger generation

Without brain health, you do not have health.

CONTENTS

CONTENTS

FOREWORD

One of my most recent motivating and exciting adventures has been honoring my commitment to enhance brain performance in Navy SEALs—a select group of military service members dedicated to being at the top of their game in all areas of performance. When I received the letter below from Morgan, I thought what better message to open my book than words from an elite performer. I hope they inspire you to take the challenge of achieving higher brain performance this very day and every day forward.

> Advances in modern medicine, science, and exercise physiology have taken our athletes to accomplishments that ten years ago were considered impossible. Usain Bolt ran faster than any human alive at the Olympic games. Mark Inglis climbed Mount Everest on two prosthetic legs. We are growing stronger, and going faster, longer, and higher than ever before.
>
> Do you realize that the winner of a contest whether it is physical or mental is the one that has endured the most pain in training? The champions of the world are the ones that accept the idea that no matter the cost they will sacrifice everything to win. Champions want to be champions, and winners are winners no matter what they are doing at the time. How far can we take the ability of our brains if we actually focused on training it like we do our bodies?
>
> My visit at the Center for BrainHealth taught me many things. One, that anyone can think smarter. Two, you can join the fight

sharper than before. Three—none more important than this—I will not fail, and I can be better, stronger, and smarter. Why? Because it's up to me, and I will succeed.

—Morgan Luttrell, Navy SEAL

INTRODUCTION

When I say, "You can increase your brain performance," people stare at me, doubtful that this could be true. It is not surprising that many would challenge the claim and believe it to be false hype.

New brain science discoveries show that individuals, young and old, can, indeed, increase their intelligence.[1-7] As a cognitive neuroscientist and founder and chief director of the Center for BrainHealth at The University of Texas at Dallas, I strive to uncover how the brain best learns and reasons, rebounds and repairs after injury, and builds resilience against decline. The goal: to maximize the amazing potential of our most vital organ—the brain.

My research and scientific discoveries have shown that most everyone can increase their intellectual capital and maximize their cognitive potential.[8-15] What does that mean for you? Simply put, you can control the destiny of your brain. You can mold your brain's frontal lobe, the epicenter of your intelligence, to grow your brainpower.

Do you want to:

- start thinking smarter today?
- learn to avoid habits that drain your cognitive potential?
- strengthen your fluid intelligence continually?
- recognize that memory lapses may not be the chief thief robbing you of your highest level of mental productivity and cognitive creativity?
- advance your capacity to be an agent of change?

The answer to each of these is—a Know Brainer. By learning how to incorporate new brain science into your daily life, you can develop the mental agility necessary to help solve the complexities of the issues you face today and the unknown ones of the future. I will guide you to improve cognitive capacity and increase your peak performance and intellectual capital.

The Limitless Frontier of Cognitive Discovery

For the past thirty years, my life has been dedicated to discovering ways to optimize brain health by applying rapidly emerging innovations to make a difference in people's lives. Through my ongoing research with a host of populations—including but not limited to healthy teens and adults; people who have suffered traumatic brain injuries such as a concussion or stroke; those with brain diseases such as Alzheimer's and other forms of dementia; and children diagnosed with autism and ADHD—I have been struck by two key findings:

- The brain's frontal lobe unequivocally contributes to building resilience, to regaining cognitive function, and to retraining the brain to maximize its extraordinary power.
- It typically takes twenty to forty years or more for scientific discoveries to trickle down to meaningfully benefit human life.

And this is why I am writing this book.

None of us can afford to let our brains decline—not even for a day. You would not accept that for your heart, eyes, or lungs, so why allow such slippage for your most valued internal asset?

If you fail to harness the incredible potential of your brain, you are inhibiting your success. You are, in essence, going backward instead of forging a blazing trail to increased productivity and boundless performance.

Our life span only continues to grow as the twenty-first century proceeds. A health-care policy journal predicts an average American life span of eighty-six years for a man and ninety-three years for a woman by mid-century[16]—more than a decade longer than today's life expectancy—a mere forty years from now. This poses numerous ethical questions. When asked, people tend to respond that they desire to live as long as they have a healthy mind, since a robust and high-functioning brain is considered the very cornerstone of a satisfactory quality of life. Surprisingly, though, the steps to improve cognitive brain function are at least a generation and a half behind what has been achieved for heart health. Significantly more needs to be done to achieve a brain health span that more closely aligns with our body's new life span. This is why brain fitness should become your personal goal.

I have dedicated my life to discovering how the brain best absorbs complex information, learns to think strategically, and innovates at its optimal level. I am determined to help people increase and maximize their brainpower.

Why the Frontal Lobe?

This book will revolutionize how you think and use your brain's frontal lobe to solve the complexities you meet each day. Your frontal lobe is the part of the brain responsible for planning, decision making, judgment, and other executive functions. You will become keenly aware of new brain discoveries regarding which frontal lobe brain habits might obstruct clear thinking and which ones could facilitate your capacity to think smarter rather than harder, day in and day out. You will learn how to build a more robust cognitive capacity, how to process information deeply and insightfully, and how to develop strategic thinking to continually upgrade your realized potential.

One is never too young or too old to commit to a brain health plan that challenges the brain's capacity to think smarter. It requires concerted and continual efforts to achieve robust frontal lobe function since each generation comes to the table with different strengths and vulnerabilities. And while there is almost no area that one cannot improve with repeated practice and proper use, the choice of what to focus on may make a difference.

Our cognitive brain health declines because we let it. We are complicit in our own brain decline by failing to keep our frontal lobe as fit as we can and should, by not adopting and incorporating healthy brain habits that daily promote dynamic and flexible thinking, and by not taking full advantage of all our brains have to offer. It is unsettling how much brain potential is lost due to neglect and improper maintenance. **When your brain-power decreases it costs you dearly. Habitual low brain performance costs an estimated $100 trillion to our gross domestic product.**[17]

The hopeful part is that science is revealing that certain brain functions, such as problem solving, synthesizing big ideas, and innovative thinking, can actually improve with advancing age,[18-22] but only if we keep these functions fine-tuned. You can play a role in slowing the rate of deterioration of many cognitive brain functions—such as difficulty with new learning brought about by lack of confidence and practice—regardless of your age.

What brain value are you willing to lose this year? Or will you take the necessary steps to experience brain gain? Become a master of your own cognitive destiny. Increase your productivity, enhance your success, maximize your potential, and boost your bottom line. Don't overthink it—there is no downside to thinking more efficiently, more clearly, and smarter.

For additional tools and tips visit www.makeyourbrainsmarter.com.

SECTION I

DISCOVER THE FRONTAL LOBE FRONTIER

CHAPTER 1

YOUR BRAIN, YOUR PRODUCTIVITY

I magine you are a nine-year-old having difficulty in school. You cannot concentrate for extended periods of time. You have trouble staying on task and, frankly, you are bored in the classroom.

You take an IQ test and are branded "average." At the early age of nine, your potential is impacted, squelched by mere words, and you are labeled as mediocre and not smart. How do you feel? Limited? Uninspired? Hopeless?

For years, this label haunts you, and your worries of being a failure grow stronger and stronger. Until one day in your twenties, you realize that you are most certainly not average—you are actually smart, and even more capable than most colleagues around you. Fast-forward thirty years, and you are a successful, innovative executive who exudes creativity and brilliant entrepreneurial skills. Despite your extraordinary achievements and unparalleled accomplishments, you still see the ghost of the early label; you think again of yourself as that nine-year-old who was deemed destined for mediocrity. Millions worldwide share this same story.

The idea that intelligence is innate—something that we are born with that cannot be altered or changed—has been deeply ingrained in conventional wisdom for almost a hundred years. Intelligence Quotient (IQ) testing remains a chief basis to determine different levels of education, potential for jobs and leadership positions, and roles in the military. The only thing that has not changed with time is the definition of intelligence. Until now.

> Sadly, when it comes to issues of the brain, many of our thoughts and ideas are outdated and backward.

The brain is our most important and widely used organ, yet it is the most neglected. You do not have to feel as if nothing can be done to improve your brain function and productivity. Your brain can be changed; it is up to you. Your brain's ability to grow and rewire itself is referred to as neuroplasticity in the science community. This means that your brain is essentially plastic, moldable, transformable, pliable, flexible, resilient, and shapable. You can strengthen cognitive brain function and brain reserves at every stage of life—even into late life.[1-3] My goal is to inspire **you** to invest in your greatest **asset** and natural **resource**—your own brain—continually.

> Your brain is the most modifiable part of your whole body, and you can rewire your brain by how you use it every single day.

How important would you say **your** brain is to your productivity? We can agree that we could not do much without our brainpower, but, admittedly, much that we are doing (and failing to do) may actually take a detrimental toll on our capacity to achieve our maximum brain potential.

People often ask me, "So what should I be doing to keep my brain healthy?" When I tell them my recommendations, they do not always like what they hear. There are three reasons for this:

1. **There is not a simple formula.** We always want something easy to do, like a certain number of puzzles to complete each day or a magic pill to take, to make us think smarter and keep our brain healthy. But a simple formula or exercise does not have a substantial and lasting impact on such a complex organ as our brain.
2. **We are creatures of habit.** We routinely rely on automatic, lower-level ways to take in, understand, and recall new information instead of using the amazing synthesizing capacity of our brains. We pride ourselves when remem-

bering information near perfectly in its original form wl...
we should be thoughtfully processing and reshaping it to
be creative thinkers. When we perform tasks by rote, our
brain's connections are not continually strengthened. In
fact, rote behavior is rotting our brain potential.

3. **It takes effort.** Our brain has to work hard to transform
ideas from content we're absorbing . . . into novel concepts and approaches. The good news is that the more you
practice deeper thinking, the easier and more efficient your
brain operates when taking on more effortful thinking.[4-7]
When you challenge your brain, you will be motivated to
achieve new heights.

**We each want to live a long life, but only if we still have our minds function-
ing and are able to make our own decisions. And to do so requires commitment to proper brain workouts—not
brain burnouts! To think smarter, you
need to learn brain habits to pursue.**

Brain science is one of the fastest
growing and most prolific fields of
discovery, largely because there is so
much to learn. Advances in new brain
imaging technology are making it possible to view brain changes in real time.
However, brain science is still at least

> New brain science
> discoveries show that
> individuals, young and old,
> can indeed increase their
> intelligence.

twenty years behind heart health. We even know more about space travel
and the universe than we do about the brain. Typically, once discoveries are
made about the brain through scientific research, it can take at least twenty
to forty years before the findings trickle down to change medical practices,
advance policy, and improve lives. But our own brains cannot wait that long.

Our brains cannot wait even a day. The
losses will continually accrue, and may
one day be too great to overcome. I am
determined to change that. In truth,
you can ramp up your mental capacity
and build your brain to think smarter
than it does today. I will show you how.

> We've learned more about
> the brain in the past ten
> years than in all previous
> years combined.

There are two critical pieces of information that are the foundation of this book. I briefly introduced the first—neuroplasticity—but want to expand upon that term here. The term "neuroplasticity" is derived from the root words "neuron" and "plastic." A neuron refers to the nerve cells in our brain. The word "plastic," as defined by Merriam-Webster's dictionary, means capable of being molded or modeled, capable of adapting to varying conditions. Neuroplasticity refers to the potential that the brain has to reorganize and rewire by birthing new neurons and creating new neural pathways.

Several decades ago scientists still widely believed that each individual was born with all the brain cells he or she would ever have and that the potential to develop new brain connections ended in adolescence. Recently neuroscientists have disproven both of these widely held beliefs. Every person can positively influence their brain's capacity to generate new brain cells and build connections in his or her own brain.[8–12]

Understanding neuroplasticity has transformed the scientific field. During the earliest stages of my career, I was intrigued and baffled by the idea that intellectual functioning was fixed. Over and over again, I have seen individuals who have manifested gains with training—healthy individuals, individuals with a brain injury, or individuals who had been diagnosed with brain disease. These individuals defied what I was first taught early in my career. The notion that brain change or brain repair is limited by age, the amount of time since injury, disease, and scale of severity has been proven false thanks to neuroplasticity.

> The brain can grow, change, rewire, repair, and heal itself continually. What hope!

The second pivotal piece of this book is the significant emphasis placed on the brain's frontal lobe. You'll learn more about the importance of this critical brain region in the next chapter, but I have discovered specific ways to expand our brain's cognitive potential by capitalizing and challenging our brain's frontal lobe. We are often complicit in our own brain decline because we don't keep our frontal lobe as fit as we can and should; we do not adopt and incorporate healthy brain habits, and we fail to take full advantage of what our brains have to offer.

The key to investing in your brain now and your cognitive reserve for the future lies largely within your remarkable frontal lobe and its deep connections to other brain areas, as well as ceasing many of the brain habits that work against healthy frontal lobe function. It is critical to adopt habits that **engage** rather than **engulf** your frontal lobe, helping you establish strong mental reserves that allow you to rethink and revamp your environment to better support your brain's health.

What happens today is a paradox: we are working longer hours in school, at home and at the office; yet, qualitatively, we are less mentally productive than we

> Overuse of Brain = Underutilized Potential

should be—a clear case where more is not better. As a society, we deeply value a strong work ethic and associate hard-charging, nonstop working with greater productivity. This incongruity between time worked and output seems like a contradiction and is hard to fathom. In reality, the news should be a relief.

What matters is the quality of the product that emanates from a brain in the "zone," not an exhausted brain that is battling through piles of endless to-dos. Think about an athlete who trains and trains to run a marathon. He runs in the mornings and trains again in the evenings. He believes the harder he runs, the better shape he will be in to complete the 26.2-mile race. But the body, like the brain, has its limits. Several weeks into training, the athlete experiences severe pain. A doctor diagnoses the problem as a stress fracture due to too much strain from exercise on the particular body part. Too much of a good thing is not a great thing. The brain can be overworked, just as the body can. With the brain there is always a trade-off, a balance to be reached.

To capture the linkage between our cognitive brain potential and productivity and our financial wherewithal, I coined the term "brainomics"; this addresses the:

- high economic costs of low brain performance.
- immense economic benefits from maximum brain performance.

Brainomics represents the attainable benefit of your richest natural resource—for personal, professional, and global gain. Increasing brainpower by even small degrees will produce immense tangible and rewarding intellectual returns on investment. For example, economists have determined that the high economic burden of stalled or low brain performance (low educational attainment) currently costs an estimated $100 trillion to our national gross domestic product (GDP) bottom line.[13]

Failing to close the gap between your brain potential and your actual performance costs you personally; it costs you professionally; it costs your family; it costs your company; and it is detrimental to your overall brain health. In short, habitual low brain performance takes its toll on your capacity to perform and maintain a high level and has a significant negative impact on your bottom line.

> You will see the greatest return on investment for the attention you give to your greatest natural resource— your brain.

Put yourself in the shoes of the following individuals who revealed important brain lessons that contradicted previously widely held views. These lessons significantly benefited their own personal and financial bottom lines, as well as those whose lives depend on them and the companies for which they work.

Myth Buster Case 1: Once memory starts to slip, a career is near its end.

Phil was afraid that he should be winding down his medical practice—not because he wanted to, but because he felt his brain was telling him he needed to. At sixty-two, he felt that he could not keep all the relevant information about his patients in his head from visit to visit—a skill in which he had always prided himself for decades. His self-doubts were put to rest when he had a BrainHealth Physical, a unique comprehensive assessment that establishes an individualized profile of cognitive performance in pivotal areas of higher-order mental functioning (you will learn more about this in chapter 3). Reassuringly, when tested, he performed extraordinarily high on intellectual skills of synthesizing, constructing abstracted meanings, and generating innovative solutions to problems—skills that are vital to providing quality medical care, skills that rely heavily on healthy frontal lobe functions. Phil's immediate memory was average but nothing else about his cognitive status was average. He demonstrated astute insights and deeply reasoned thoughts that were more vital to his professional cognitive demands. His *extraordinary frontal lobe function, not just his memory,* provided the fuel needed to ensure sound life-and-death medical decisions that he had to make daily for excellent patient care.

Brainomics: Abstract thinking and problem solving are core intellectual processes that reflect a robust mind, more so than simple straightforward memory. If Phil had retired at sixty-two, it would have been a devastating loss to his practice and to the beneficiaries of his practice—his patients. Some five years later, he is still at the top of his game, staying abreast of new treatment offerings, improving his brain health by his continuous complex thinking, and boosting both his community's and his own personal well-being and financial bottom line every day.

Myth Buster Case 2: Medications alone are the best first-line treatments to help students with attention deficit/hyperactivity disorder (ADHD) to improve their learning.

Fourteen-year-old Todd had always been successful in elementary school, but in middle school his test and homework scores began to drop with no relief in sight. His declining performance was not due to lack of effort but because of his maladaptive strategies to overcome his attention deficit/hyperactivity disorder (ADHD).

"I would spend hours trying to help him complete his homework assignments," his mother said. "It wasn't that he didn't want to learn, but he quickly became overwhelmed by the massive amounts of information. He was trying to remember so many facts."

"I struggled with reading problems and writing out my answers," Todd said. "I needed something to change in order to improve my test-taking abilities and reading comprehension."

After ten sessions of brain training, where he learned how to engage in top-down processing by pursuing bigger concepts instead of bottom-up learning, which focuses on rote fact memorization, Todd began to construct abstract meanings from lessons and generate innovative solutions to problems. Soon he completed his homework assignments in one-fifth the time, and his grades returned to his A-level potential.

"With the training, Todd felt empowered and equipped to more effectively assimilate, manage, and utilize information," his father said.

"After training, I thought of my assignments in a different way. Todd said. "I approached homework more inspired, seeing how I could think bigger thoughts myself and break down assignments step by step. Learning became easier, and I was able to write more creatively. To top it off, my grades got better in all of my classes."

Brainomics: Strategic reasoning that involves transformed ideas rather than rote learning may enhance attentiveness for students with ADHD beyond what medication can attain alone. For some individuals, *medication may become unnecessary*. Indeed, Todd was able to stop the medication as his study skills improved, and he no longer needed the medication to help him focus. Just imagine the cost savings from elevating educational attainment level, controlling tutor costs, and reducing the need for medication costs. Most of all, some four years later, Todd has regained his confidence as a learner and innovative thinker and has set high expectations for himself as he prepares for college and a career as a statesman.

Myth Buster Case 3: The more exacting our memory, the more brainpower we will experience/exhibit.

Susan, a twenty-two-year-old, mostly A student through school, was hired right out of college as a project coordinator tasked with managing minute details and orchestrating schedules. After three years she was stuck in the same position and was never given an opportunity to advance her career. Why? She was consistently valued and rewarded for her keen attention to details. She was never challenged to exercise her innovative mind to offer fresh ideas and directions. She was being trained to be a perfect robot of ideas—taking in and spitting back data like a computer. Her creative mind was not stimulated so that it could grow.

In Susan's case, her remarkable ability to master details and information led to a great starting opportunity at a wonderful company. Unfortunately, without being intellectually challenged to create novel ideas and see the big picture, she was left bored and frustrated. Her position required prioritizing key decisions to be made, but because all the details and steps seemed equally important, she could not weed out and pare down the data to the essentials. Since Susan was not privy to the bigger goals, she was not learning how the pieces fit into the whole, leaving her feeling stuck, inadequate, and not integral to the overall mission of the company.

Brainomics: Young professionals are burning out and not able to contribute to futuristic paths because they are continually stuck in habitual rote learning. They are *building a brain that retains high volumes of data, but not a brain that can think critically, get out of status-quo mentality, and figure out new paths and solutions*. Educational systems across the country reinforce the importance of memorization and fact learning. Corporations must now provide the proper training environment where young professionals can learn to properly acquire and expand their creative potential, otherwise their potential will stagnate as it did in Susan's case.

> Quality over quantity. It is not how much knowledge capacity you have, but how you use what you know to solve new problems and chart new directions.

There is massive turnover in young top talent, and the costs associated with hiring and training a replacement are not economical. Turnover also drains potential high performers, whose talent is underdeveloped because of inadequate opportunities and brain challenges that engage higher-level strategic thinking, weighed discernment, and dynamic problem solving.

Myth Buster Case 4: The more we use our brains, the stronger they will be.

Forty-year-old Ben, a vice president of a major corporation, was feeling taxed. He constantly pushed his brain, overloading it with information by continually exposing himself to new courses and the latest leadership books and forcing it to complete an impressive litany of tasks at one time. With a packed schedule of back-to-back meetings and a constant open-door policy, Ben felt responsible for putting out all the fires at his company. "I always thought that the harder I worked my brain, the better," he said when I first met him.

Brainomics: In fact, the conventional wisdom of "use it or lose it" has become so oversubscribed that many of us are counterproductive. We are using our brain ("overusing" may be a better word for it) in such an unruly, rampant, and superficial way that we are failing to build and strengthen a mind that intentionally determines what to pursue and what NOT to pursue. Trying to solve every problem, rather than discerning which problems to focus on and which to put aside, leaves us distracted and increases brain drain. *Overuse of your brain is progressively detrimental.* There are major trade-offs to a brain that is constantly firing on all cylinders, diminishing intellectual growth.

Your brain builds deeper connections across ideas when you can take a step back and rest; letting your brain have downtime leads to greater insights, more fruitful pursuits of the important, and deeper-level thinking.[14-15] Efficiently using your brain equals increased mental productivity and richer intellectual resources.

Myth Buster Case 5: The aging brain has lost its potential for brain plasticity—where plasticity means capacity to be modified to rebound from injury.

Aaron was CEO of his own thriving business that he'd started some fifty years before. At eighty-one he had a stroke, which resulted in aphasia—problems expressing his ideas fluently due to damage to the language hemisphere. Aaron was told that he would never be able to go back to work, due mostly to his age but also his difficulty talking, the cognitive residual from his stroke. When I saw him one and a half years later as part of my dissertation work, Aaron was severely depressed and "stuck" due to minimal mental stimulation.

I asked him what his aims were for himself, and he answered that he desperately wanted to go back to work but was told that he did not have the cognitive capacity. After assessing his ability to synthesize and absorb content meaning, I was astounded by his astute intellectual capacity to draw abstract ideas from complex information, although he conveyed this in choppy language. How was this high level of performance possible given a severe stroke at his advanced age? After all, I had learned that the aging brain had little, if any, potential to recover. His high performance belied current thinking on brain plasticity in the older brain. He absolutely had the cognitive capacity to go back to work!

With two months of training, he was back at work part-time and continued to show recovery until he passed away some five years later. His son reported that Aaron got his life back and was certainly able to make sound decisions for the company to keep it thriving.

Brainomics: Our brain retains its ability to rebound from injury later in life—especially if we remain mentally active. Think of the cost burden of keeping Aaron disabled because of age, the perceived residuals of stroke, and the belief that the brain could not continue to recover one year after it had been damaged. This is not about incurring increased rehabilitative costs; instead, it's about taking advantage of the real-life cognitive repair that can take place in familiar life-work stimulating environments. Clearly, the positive brainomics of boosting brainpower into late life can have major cost savings. Aaron was likely able to return to work after his stroke because he'd built formidable cognitive reserves by challenging his brain through complex thinking all his life.

Aaron and his story inspired me to take a strong stance against the negative view of brain repair based on chronological age; I was so encouraged by his robust brain health that one of my first published papers shared his story. Aaron personified the immense potential of the aging mind to regain cognitive function despite a brain injury.

When people ask me where I think we will make the greatest impact in brain research, I quickly say it will not only be in people *with* brain injury or brain disease; we will make even more positive strides in normal, healthy individuals from teens to twentysomethings, to baby boomers, and for sure into late life for those nearing one hundred years of age. Only recently have scientists, physicians, and the general public begun to address brain fitness in healthy people. Why? Because we only thought brain issues were related to losses that emerged from brain injuries or brain diseases. In the absence of disease, it's essential to detect your own cognitive vulnerabilities, accept what cannot be changed (such as the speed with which you learn new information at older ages), and boost your brainpower in core areas to achieve optimal mental profitability that will powerfully benefit every aspect of your life.

> The impact of subpar brain performance (and even brain decline) can be felt most dramatically on your personal bottom line and sense of well-being.

The issue of how your brain thinks (cognition) at all ages is so vital to our nation that you cannot put off your brain's health any longer. But conventional wisdom says "If it ain't broke, don't fix it," leading many to believe if something is working adequately well, leave it alone. **For your brain, mediocrity and status quo are hurting your quest to think and be smarter, longer.**

> Your brainpower can be harnessed to increase creativity and mental productivity.

With healthier brain function, you will remain productive longer and continue to make significant contributions to the well-being and productivity of your family, your community, and our nation. Time is of the essence. Failure to reach your brain potential and declines in brain capacity grow increasingly worse with advancing age. It is up to you to take control of your mental command center and make improved thinking an attainable mission.

Investing in your brain's future, and specifically your brain's frontal lobe, is critical because this elaborate system is the control center for your thinking potential.[16–21] Your complex frontal lobe network, as you will learn in the next chapter, serves as your brain's unimpeachable commander in chief. Your frontal lobe must be efficient, productive, and dynamically flexible to maximize your brain potential and your personal potential.

What robs you of your mental productivity? I suspect you might respond as many do:

- Too many emails to get through
- Too much information to absorb
- Massive demands from others
- Too long a to-do list
- Constant interruptions
- No downtime
- Lack of sleep
- Rampant distractions
- Mindless and unfocused meetings
- Fast pace of changes
- Too many late night events
- A mind that will not turn off

Become an executive to your own brain health and you will reap decreases in illness and absenteeism, reductions in stress and brain fatigue, and increases in your profitability. The United States has recently witnessed a notable decline in innovation, and it is facing stronger economic competition from other nations. But any country can dramatically raise its gross domestic product as the brainpower of its citizens increases.

The math is simple: even the most marginal rate of individual improvement in brain capacity will have exponentially positive impacts when multiplied across populations. The upside of brainomics focuses on increasing personal and society brain net worth, thereby making the world a more innovative, thought-filled, dynamically visionary, and profitable place. Are you up to the challenge? There is no limit to your brain's potential.

Know Brainers

1. Brainomics: incremental increases in brainpower will have an exponential impact on your bottom line.
2. We have learned more about the brain and its

capability to be strengthened and repaired in the past ten years than in all previous years combined.

3. Increase or decrease your brainpower: You decide. Your brain changes from moment to moment depending on how you use it.

4. Maximizing human cognitive potential requires regular investments from an individual.

5. Age can be an asset for brain gain in keystone cognitive capacities.

6. The conventional wisdom of "use it or lose it" is driving down the net worth of our brains.

CHAPTER 2

FRONTAL LOBE FITNESS RULES

Why does frontal lobe power make you think smarter—not harder?

When were you the smartest?

How would you define being smart?

What do you worry about the most in terms of brain function?

Why is synthesizing meaning more vital to solving the complex everyday life problems than remembering specific facts?

What cognitive habits do you need to break to become a flexible thinker?

Why is novel thinking greater fuel for robust cognitive function than thinking in routine ways?

What is fluid intelligence, and is it the same as IQ?

What are the limitations of the saying "use or lose it" when applied to your brainpower?

Why is complex thinking good for your brain's neurons?

One of the greatest accomplishments of the past century is the doubling of the human life span. Unfortunately, our brain span has not been increased at all. When do you think your brain was operating at its peak performance? It is important for you to pause for a moment to think about the age you felt you were in your optimal mental zone. Write that age down. I want you to write it down before continuing to read on because you will be asked to look back on this age as you learn more about how you can think smarter—longer.

> ## I was sharpest at age _____.

I ask this question frequently because it always amazes me how people respond. Invariably, they throw out ages at least ten to twenty years younger than they are currently. "When I was fifty," say some, while others say, "When I was twenty-five," and still others, "When I was six years old"—all are frequent ages that I hear.

The typical reaction reflects the assumption that our best brain years are behind us:

- I was smartest twenty years ago, when I could remember phone numbers without a second thought.
- I was smartest when I was in college, when I could absorb facts like a sponge.
- I was smartest when I was in my thirties, with intellectual energy that never waned.
- I was smartest when I was three years old; every day my knowledge increased dramatically.

> Most people believe their best brain years are in the past. Grim thought!

Then I ask people, if you think you were smarter back then, could you perform what you are doing today, say, some twenty or thirty years ago? Not likely. Then why do we think we were sharper back then and not now?

It is appalling that in a world where more people are living to be older than ever before, aging is still seen as a form of disease. We have grown to fully expect that cognitive decline is an inevitable consequence of aging, even though the majority of seniors aged eighty-five and older manifest a potential for well-preserved intellect, capacity for new learning, and sound decision making.[1-3] We live believing our best brain years are in the past. What a depressing thought.

People often ask: How do I know if I am thinking sharper or if my thinking is stilted or stalled? How do I know if I am just plain losing it? Do annoying memory glitches mean I am losing my brainpower?

Ask yourself these questions to help you determine if your brainpower is where it should and could be:

1. Am I able to weigh the risks and benefits of decisions?
   For example: Would you feel comfortable weighing the pros and cons of taking a new job?

2. Am I able to come up with creative solutions to problems?
   For example: Do you know where to go to find the information needed to creatively solve a problem? And do you know when you have enough information to come to a workable resolution?

3. Am I a flexible thinker?
   For example: Are you comfortable departing from traditional modes of thought—from the known to the unknown?

If you answered no to any one of these questions, it is time to tune up your frontal lobe capacity.

Imagine a day without the ability to recognize the need for and embrace change, without the facility to reflect from a broader perspective and manage stressful situations, without the understanding of friendship and managing one's emotions, without being capable of identifying meaningful personal goals and making sound decisions to achieve them. A day without the ability to reason, execute plans, or imagine different options. Sound impossible?

To me, this seems to be a day without the use of efficient, functional frontal lobes—at least the prefrontal cortex and its intricate connections.

Take Jeremy, an extremely bright, talented, and creative fiftysomething who was struggling to manage his workload, his stress level, and his emotions. At first glance, he seemed to excel at being a dedicated worker with a positive and upbeat attitude, pursuing excellence. His career thrived on those admirable characteristics, but after further conversations, he confessed that he struggled to stay on task—any task, big or small. When given an assignment from his boss, Jeremy could rarely complete it to the level of his potential, instead getting bogged down by not knowing where to begin or what to pursue. In the end, he would shut down and turn in mediocre work just to get the assignment off his plate.

Upon assessment, it was clear that Jeremy was not struggling with motivation or ambition. Instead, his frontal lobe was failing him: it was performing inadequately, which led to even more stress, more brain drain, and lower performance.

Your frontal lobe is your higher-order cognitive command center responsible for novel thinking. It represents nearly a third of our entire brain and is intimately involved in orchestrating our capacity to reason, think abstractly, solve novel problems, flexibly deploy mental resources to update information, and generate insightful ideas.

Car rental companies knew what they were doing when they refused to loan cars to those younger than age twenty-five; raw statistics exposed the fact that young adult brains were not making rational and sound driving decisions. Brain science has now revealed that the frontal lobe is not fully developed until the late twenties.[4-6] From early adolescence to young adulthood, the frontal lobe, and the intricate connections between it, are undergoing dramatic functional and structural changes that remodel the brain's complex connectivity and advance its capacity to engage in integrated, reasoned, and high-level thinking.[7]

Anatomically, the frontal lobe, as illustrated below, sits in the front of the brain, just above your eyes in your skull. I adopt the practice of using the term "frontal lobe," as do many cognitive neuroscientists, when discussing higher-order cognitive functions commonly linked to the prefrontal cortex and its complex connections.

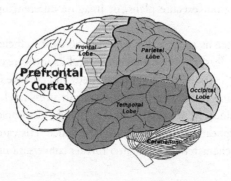

When engaged, frontal lobe brain functions serve to integrate various processes that are essential to independent thinking and decision making.[8–12] Even seemingly simple tasks rely heavily on the frontal lobe working in tandem with other brain networks—interpreting the message from a book or a movie, conveying important ideas in an email, planning and orchestrating a holiday party, or even mapping a route to a new destination. Complex frontal lobe connections are essential to helping us thrive personally and professionally in a rapidly changing world.

New research findings reveal that the road to thinking *smarter* appears to lead to the brain's intricate frontal lobe networks. The dynamic power of the frontal lobe is what allows you to think smarter and deeper every year of life. So much of what you need to accomplish daily is complex and new, requiring heavy lifting by your frontal lobe. Because of its unique abilities, many refer to the frontal lobe as the *sedes sapientiae,* the "seat of wisdom."[13–14] The power of your frontal lobe integrity is what separates you from all other life forms. **Harnessing that power will lead to increased brain potential, maximized brain efficiency, enhanced productivity, and enriched creativity and innovation.**

High-level thinking skills that you so often take for granted, such as figuring out what investment to make, what home to buy, or what job to pursue, emanate from the power of your frontal lobe functions. Those who study cognition often refer to these complex mental challenges as "fluid intelligence"—how dynamically and flexibly individuals use what they know and how they apply learning to new contexts. Fluid intelligence is manifested through the ability to deal with new and uncertain situations and to plan futuristically to solve problems in systematic ways. In contrast, "crystallized intelligence" refers to how much one knows and how much experience one has—that is, how much knowledge has been accrued.

Fluid intelligence relies heavily on the integrity of the prefrontal cor-

> Achieve your brain's potential to solve the most complex problems you face daily.

> Your prefrontal cortex serves as your personal CEO.

21

tex, and many cognitive neuroscientists refer to fluid intelligence skills as executive functions.[15] The core executive functions are: inhibition[16-19] (e.g., blocking distractions), switching[20-21] (e.g., toggling back and forth between tasks), working memory (e.g. active maintenance and manipulation of information), and flexibility (e.g., changing and updating old knowledge). The integration of these specific processes works in concert to achieve the complex and multidimensional cognitive functions of problem solving, reasoning, planning, and abstracting.[22-24] Fluid intelligence allows you to organize your day and successfully manage the large volumes of information confronting you each moment.

> Novel thinking keeps your brain thriving to support the cognitive demands of a fast-changing culture.

Exploring the best path to increase your brain's net worth—whether you are in your thirties, fifties, or eighties—requires continually strengthening your fluid intelligence. But how do you do that? You will learn more in later chapters, but achieving this goal boils down to **constantly** and dynamically managing, monitoring, and problem solving when faced with new situations, context, ideas, or issues. Fluid intelligence allows you to assimilate and reconcile disparate pieces of information, which you have acquired over your lifetime—perhaps some even this very day—in novel ways to create something **new.** Fluid intelligence skills are called upon when you engage in the ability to manipulate, monitor, and change your thinking in order to deal with stressful contexts or uncertain futures.[25-32] The goal is to repeatedly improve plans, ideas, or actions based on up-to-the-minute information. For example: Will you flexibly apply this book's new recommendations to your life? It is challenging and requires consistent effort to consciously tap into and train the power of your frontal lobe to change your ways.

So, how do you know if you are enlisting and challenging your novel-thinking potential? Ask yourself which side of the fence you stand on these questions:

Do you have the same dinner guests repeatedly?	Do you invite an unexpected guest to change up the conversation?
Do your regular gatherings with colleagues, friends, or family discuss the same predictable topics?	Do your gatherings always have an interesting new topic to discuss?
Do you express the same ideas to convey your stance on issues over and over?	Do you continually attempt to see things from a new perspective when you discuss a topic?
Do you adamantly resist using new technology, such as a new cell phone?	Do you stay open to moving from old to new technology?
Do your emails sound the same? Do you send cards following predictable traditions?	Do you think of creative ideas and unique timing to convey personal messages?
Do you stop short and only complete the task asked of you by your spouse, relative, or boss without reflecting on the process?	Do you add your own thinking to the task at hand or even try to offer new approaches to improve the outcome or solve an unexpected problem?

If you answered yes to the questions on the left, then you are not harnessing the power of your frontal lobe to achieve your greatest potential. But you can.

It is becoming increasingly important to strengthen your fluid intelligence and integrative frontal lobe functions to deal with an unknown future. The ability to succeed at every stage of life—whether in school, in the workplace, in retirement, or in marriage—largely depends on fluid intelligence rather than on how much you know or what your IQ score was at some point in time.

Success = flexible mental resources

Think about it. Success is highly related to the ability to dynamically draw upon and flexibly deploy mental resources to solve new problems, recognize aspects that need to be changed, know when to act on new insights or serendipities, and discern how to resist temptation to do something that would be irrelevant or regrettable. Your frontal lobe and its complex networks have far-reaching influences on almost all major complex mental activities,[33–35] including how to use the latest technology, learn the skills required for a new job or promotion, or develop an impressive presentation or organize a memorable birthday celebration. Those are just a few examples.

Central Command

Your frontal lobe sits in a privileged position as the brain's central command headquarters, linking information back and forth across other brain regions. This elaborate brain communication network guides behaviors by managing incoming information and associating it with existing knowledge stored across brain regions. Your frontal lobe has the vastest neural network and the most reciprocal interconnections with other brain structures.[36–40] This underscores its superiority in controlling our most complex and abstract higher-order thinking capacity. In other words, your frontal lobe power allows you to monitor, manage, and manipulate how you successfully coordinate your day, acquire and apply new things you've learned, and think futuristically.

> Executive functions are more important for everyday life performance and independence than your IQ or intelligence quotient.

Paradoxically and intriguingly, recent brain imaging studies show that frontal lobe functions are the last to develop in the brain and the first to decline.[41–43] The intricate neural circuitry of the prefrontal cortex is *the* control center for complex cognitive functions,[44–45] and it is vitally important to focus on frontal lobe development.

Frontal lobe functions are integral to managing and orchestrating the complex matters of everyday life during all stages of life. For the most part, individuals only think of being concerned about brain health in terms of injury or disease, where you can certainly see more vividly the detrimental impact of impaired frontal lobe functions. However, strong frontal lobe

> Everyone needs to invest in his or her own brain health as early and as long as possible.

functions are crucial in healthy development from adolescence until late life. When people learn what I research—how to maximize human cognitive potential—they say, "I don't need that [aka brain health] yet!"

Much research has focused on the enormous importance of frontal lobe functions in developing youth. But principles gleaned from frontal lobe development in youth are applicable to our brains even as we grow very old. Take the principles from the groundbreaking work of Drs. Adele Diamond and Kathleen Lee's research lab[46] at the University of British Columbia and BC Children's' Hospital in Vancouver, showing that:

- increasing frontal lobe cognitive functions elevates the brain potential of youth at greatest risk for academic failure; e.g., those from lower-income families and those with ADHD.
- in order to maintain gains, frontal lobe skills must be continually utilized and challenged.
- proper cognitive training increases frontal lobe fitness without medication.
- training to utilize complex frontal lobe functions is linked to more generalized benefits in additional untrained areas, whereas training of specific cognitive processes leads to narrow gains and minimal, if any, transfer.
- also intriguing is that stress, loneliness, and lack of physical fitness are associated with low frontal lobe functioning.

Diamond and Lee's work perfectly captures the relationship between frontal lobe functions and the real world: "As go frontal lobe EFs [executive function skills]—so goes school readiness and academic achievement."

I could modify their statement to read: "If frontal lobe executive function skills increase or decrease—so does job performance, family and home management, and personal discernment and decision making for the rest of our life."

Your frontal lobe prowess requires molding in youth with increasingly more disciplined sharpening for the rest of your lives.

Indeed, the above statement applies at every stage of life, yet adults all too often stop thinking of their brains after academic training is over, typically in their twenties. How could you neglect your brain from your twenties on? The answer is you cannot.

The current dilemma, however, is that a mature level of frontal lobe thinking is not a given, regardless of numerical age. Many young people today are failing to develop the full potential of their frontal lobe and critical thinking capacity, as you will learn later. If not given proper training, or allowance to experience some risks, or adequate opportunities to stretch thinking, the ability to perform sound decision making may stall and even fail to develop.

Combine this news of late-developing brain maturation with scientific discoveries that the brain's complex connectivity begins to decline in the forties with the first losses in the frontal brain regions. This paints a pretty dim picture revealing only, at most, twenty years of prime brain function. Can you imagine only having prime thinking for a mere twenty years? I can't. **Adults are living too long without developing, strengthening, and maintaining our amazing frontal lobe potential.** You can have the luxury of utilizing your frontal lobe power longer and building cognitive reserves, if you exercise the core capacities continually. Remember: the brain can continue to grow and change throughout your life.

> The more your cognitive function declines, the faster you slide. Apply the brakes!

Cognitive decline is not a given but is due, in large part, to your own behavior. The adoption of the pervasive laissez-faire attitude of putting your brain on automatic pilot increases the likelihood of mental slippage. Are your days mundane, filled with routine? The failure to pursue being a change maker sentences you to uncontrolled brain losses. Wouldn't you like to avoid this slippery slope?

Fortunately, large degrees of decline in certain cognitive areas may

> Be empowered: You can mold your brain to think sharper to increase your brainpower.

be avoided if you proactively target strategic thinking, especially if you strengthen your mental capital in areas of passion and expertise.[47] Doing so promotes continued stability and the growth of the key pillars needed to enhance frontal lobe brain functions.

You'll learn how to adopt and practice strategic thinking, **to enhance your brain potential.**

If the mantra "use it or lose it" is true of your brain, then today you are likely using your brain so much that you should be in a place that is beyond smart. Are you constantly pushing your brain, overloading it with information, and asking it to complete many tasks at one time? Does your brain feel like Grand Central Station during rush hour? Recall Ben from chapter 1 whose brain was constantly exposed to interruptions. What if, like Ben, you are using your brain in a detrimental way and to such an exhaustive degree that you are actually making it less efficient, less creative, and perhaps even burning it out?

Take another case of a single, forty-five-year-old communications executive with whom I recently worked. He made an appointment for an assessment to establish a benchmark of his cognitive abilities and monitor his brain and memory degeneration. He reported that as a function of his job, he is "always on" and works "twenty-four hours a day, seven days a week for 365 days a year." He never loses touch with his BlackBerry, emails during breakfast meetings, texts during lunch outings, and rarely delegates tasks to other team members. In other words, he constantly multitasks, always dividing his attention and rarely, if ever, practices gatekeeping. He overuses his brain! But he can regain control of his mental workstation and increase productivity.

> Multitasking is toxic to your brain and your health.

Multitasking, a common practice for the populace at large, is definitely robbing us of frontal lobe brainpower and reducing its fitness. It is one of the most toxic things you can do to your brain and its health. Multitasking may be a chief culprit in destroying brain cells. We have all become addicted to technology and multitasking.[48–50] But it is not a healthy addiction (learn more in chapter 4). Science demonstrates that the human brain is not wired to perform two tasks at once. Multitasking requires that the frontal lobe quickly switch back and forth between chores. This high-performance demand to

> Age is just a number. With brain age, older should be better.

smoothly switch back and forth fatigues the frontal lobe, slows efficiency, and decreases performance.[51-52]

A client of mine proudly celebrates her age and continually relies on her thinking to maximize her cognitive potential each day. At eighty-three, she is actively involved in strategic business decisions at a financial services company. Undeterred by her numeric age, she is involved in professional projects and community programs that maintain and strengthen her brain's fitness. Whereas most people set themselves up to go on automatic pilot during their last work days and retirement years, this is a bad state of affairs for the brain. **The longer we stay actively engaged in complex thinking and meaningful work, the more energized the brain is and the more cognitive reserves are being built.**

Fine-tuned brain performance is integral to a fine life. The possibilities of increasing your intellectual potential are unending in the absence of disease. Who would have ever thought that you could engineer your brain and help mold how long your mental sharpness would thrive? Of course, genetic, environmental, and social factors are also in the mix in determining your mental sharpness, but brain science reveals that neurons are literally *born* in response to complex thinking and problem solving.[53-59] Complex thinking keeps neurons healthier and more fit—just like physical exercise keeps your muscles more fit.

> Brain neurons live longer when learning is taking place.

Truly remarkable! Just think, you engineer your brain's own health by actively learning. Who said college is for the young? We need to expand our vision of education or at least promote lifelong learning courses.

Previous science writings led scientists, health professionals, and the public, in general, to believe that the brain's life span is associated with insidious and substantial declines year after year. As previously stated, **cognitive decline is happening as a result of nonaction.** Cognitive decline affects your personal and the national economic bottom line. Now is the time to spend effort on building your human cognitive capital to boost your brainomics.

> Complex thinking builds cognitive reserves and increases mental capacity.

And you can do it. If you continually challenge your frontal lobe skills, your best brain years are ahead of you. Truth is, you should be your sharpest now—if you are keeping your brain fit. Your brain has incorporated a lifetime of learning and resonant experiences that can fuel it with the additional flexibility, insight, and judgment it needs to compute effectively in today's hectic world. Prior reports that documented significant age-related declines in fluid intelligence—the ability to think flexibly, engage in abstract reasoning, and solve novel problems—are being reversed. Recent research shows that fluid intelligence is significantly modifiable, despite numeric age, for the better.[60-62]

Brain aging is not, in fact, a vexation to be avoided; rather, it is a developmental process that adds valuable perspective to the brain's existing higher-order thinking abilities. Your brain may be getting older, but if continually fine-tuned, it should also be getting more efficient. And smarter, too. In healthy brain aging, your goal should not be to look for the fountain of youth mythical elixir to return to our younger brain state. Rather, the goal should be to maintain and strengthen your brain's robustness. Keep reminding yourself, if you do not work to improve your brain, you will go backward. For your brain's well-being, you want to keep progressing. If I were to take ten or twenty years off your brain, you would beg me to have the years back because they are packed with such rich developments, that is, if you properly fostered your brain fitness. If you think brains are optimally performing in thirtysome-thing-year-olds, have them make a decision or two for you.

> Your best brain years can be in the future.

This is not to ignore the fact that as we age, certain cognitive processes show inevitable decline.[63-68] As you age, your brain:

- is slower to learn new things, such as technology; although it is still able to learn, it just takes more time,
- becomes less efficient at storing enormous volumes of new facts,
- experiences increasing numbers of annoying memory access glitches, and
- has increasing difficulty blocking out background noise.

The hopeful news is that even these declining processes can be slowed with effort and practice.[69-74]

The power behind building stronger brain connections is driven largely by how you use your brain to engage in complex and innovative thinking.[75-77] Conversely, you weaken or even lose connections when you think

> Your cognitive capacity can increase with each decade.

superficially. Consider the superior brainpower of some of the great thinkers—Albert Einstein, T. Boone Pickens, Sandra Day O'Connor, Diane Sawyer, Stephen Hawking, and Alan Greenspan. At a general level, these brainy people are thought to be the exception rather than the rule.

These magnificent minds are curious, creative, extraordinary problem solvers and futuristic thinkers. Much can be done to increase these unique abilities in all individuals, especially you, by reframing your thinking to embrace your brain's fullest intellectual potential. In thinking smarter, you can become the rule rather than the exception. Still not convinced of the immense potential you have to neuroengineer, rewire, and build your brain? Your brain changes moment to moment, depending on how you use it every day—to think, learn, create, problem solve, imagine, love, decide, and plan. And the truth is, you *can* think smarter.

> The potential to think broader, deeper, and from a higher perspective increases as you age—thanks to your frontal lobe functions.

Even more exciting is the news that brain aging can have some clear advantages when compared to the young adult brain. There are more decisive pieces to your brain puzzle as you age than speed and amount of fact recall. Certain pivotal brain functions do not have to get slowly worse and can even get better.[78-83]

I would go so far as to say that the benefits of more strategic-thinking capacity outweigh the speed and volume of a vast memory for numbers and/or facts. Sound like the lesson conveyed in "The Tortoise and the Hare"? The

> Full frontal: Engage your frontal lobe to increase brainpower.

lifelong lesson of this ageless fable holds true—slow is often a good thing, especially when it comes to pondering critical life issues.

I recently worked with two women both in the same field but with very different frontal lobe thinking patterns. Both were intelligent, hardworking, and goal oriented. The younger, with less experience, a thirty-year-old, demonstrated quick but fixed rote thinking. She did not challenge herself to develop new ideas that were not already stated or in practice based on the training materials we were reviewing. On the other hand, the fifty-year-old constantly explored, was curious about different perspectives, and made new recommendations, taking longer to ponder the major issues. The latter individual demonstrated powerful integrated reasoning capabilities and robust cognitive reserve.

Interestingly, as a society we desperately want flawless memory and are fixated on memory glitches, which are frustrating, for sure, but, as you will see in later chapters, memory remains one of the easiest skills to compensate for in the absence of injury or disease. Indeed, memory recall slows with increasing age. You will find in chapter 4 why the information that was on the tip of your tongue but eluded you when you most needed it comes to you when you are no longer searching.

> Mine your greatest natural resource—your brain.

It fascinates me how wrong we have been about the brain for so many years. Point in fact: all the aggravations of age-related memory loss, as well as losses associated with brain diseases such as Alzheimer's, were equated with brain-cell decline or failure. Up until just recently, scientists believed that brain cells were dying from birth. Now, as Caleb Finch states

> Move beyond memory as your chief brain concern.

so eloquently in the cover article for the 2001 spring edition of *USC Health* magazine,[84] "Now, it is really clear that if you don't have a specific disease that causes loss of nerve cells, then most, if not all, of the neurons remain healthy until you die." These findings change the conversation and the future for brain health. They should inspire you to take advantage of your brain's potential. They inspire me!

Your frontal lobe integrity is what allows you to live independently lon-

Live independently longer with intact brain health.

ger, not the strength of your memory capacity. My father is a perfect example of someone with an impressive memory who could not function independently at ninety years old. Dad's memory was commendable, but his frontal lobe was letting him down. He could not decide what bill to pay or what piece of mail to keep or discard. He knew exactly where every dollar he owned was in his many accounts, each with limited assets—even rainy-day funds that he kept holed away in a filing cabinet for emergency purposes. When we moved my dad from his house to an adult residence, he asked what happened to the $832 that was in the back folder in his file cabinet. He had not touched the money for more than five years, but amazingly, when we counted it, he knew down to the dollar what amount was there. He had an intact and incredible memory but was unable to manage stressful situations or his household bills and upkeep.

Memory ≠ smart

A near perfect memory is not the definition of a robust brain.

I have worked with many people with stellar memory capacities who nonetheless are not highly innovative, insightful, creative, or, for that matter, mentally productive. In fact, memory appears to work independently of strategic frontal lobe functions rather than synergistically. Would you still want a photographic memory if you knew it could hamper your higher-level thinking capacity? It can. And it does.

One of the most vivid illustrations of the link between frontal lobe capacity and everyday life success and independence was documented by the dramatic changes in cognitive facility in Phineas Gage.[85] Gage's situation dates back more than a hundred and fifty years. Gage was struck in the frontal lobe with an iron tamping bar as a result of an accidental explosion at a railroad construction site in Vermont. He regained simple cognitive functions, including memory, for his job responsibilities, enough to be able to physically return to work, but he was a changed man. Gage was unable to successfully engage in the necessary higher-order thinking skills to manage his own life, much less others he had previously overseen as their boss. He could not make simple and sound decisions or stick with plans he made. He had changed so much that the railroad company where he had previously been a model foreman refused to hire him back.

Research has shown that when regions within the frontal lobe or regions connected to the frontal lobe are damaged or not working properly, simple life tasks are difficult despite relatively intact intellectual function.[86–89] Some of the key difficulties are described as:

> Impaired frontal networks are an impediment to independent living.

- Poor insight and ability to take perspective
- Unsound judgment
- Irresponsibility
- Unreliable problem-solving skills
- Marked limitation in abstract thinking and creativity
- Rigid mental flexibility
- Fragile ability to manage emotions
- Poor management of stressful situations

My scientific discoveries[90–94] show that the clues to higher-level cognitive brain performance reside in how you engage, build, and strengthen your frontal lobe functions, including:

- Thinking strategically and futuristically
- Creating novel solutions and products
- Assimilating and reducing complex material to its absolute essence
- Constructing interpretations to improve information absorption
- Priming flashes of insight
- Updating and revising out-of-date goals and knowledge
- Identifying potential problems
- Tackling problems before they appear
- Dealing with new, uncertain circumstances
- Dynamically and flexibly shifting between information to create solutions

More attention is required to build complex strategy-based thinking, which is driven largely by your frontal lobe connections. New brain science reveals strategy-based skills are the foundational pillars that will enhance your brain edge every day and expand our own intellectual capital.[95-100]

> High-performance brain training increases frontal lobe power.

What I have found through my research is the identification of three key frontal lobe processes that are responsible for higher-order brain function: **strategic attention, integrated reasoning,** and **mental flexibility**.[101-4] In truth, very few individuals are indeed reaching their maximum cognitive potential—even executives who feel at the top of their game can improve. I challenge myself daily. I am always pursuing new ways to improve my research because each day offers a gift of new brain potential.

Making a conscious effort to properly engage complex frontal lobe functions will help you attain a higher performance level. As I delve into these pivotal areas, you will begin to understand why these multidimensional cognitive capacities are the keys to building robust frontal lobe function that will promote mental independence throughout life. Then in subsequent chapters, you will learn how to practice ways to build these prime cognitive skills.

> You can build cognitive reserves that will add years to your brain's life.

I will take you through a newly discovered, scientifically proven course designed to increase high-performing frontal lobe capacity in order to elevate your brain's control center in whichever arenas you spend your time and energy—whether you work at home, in the corporate world, or in the community. **You will come to see why frontal lobe fitness rules, no matter your generation, no matter your life's work.** You will learn ways to properly engage your frontal lobe networks to build cognitive brain reserves needed to support a long productive life. Train yourself to increase your dynamic thinking capacity by harvesting the natural integrative abilities of your frontal lobe.

> My goal: To match your brain health span to your life span.

Now I want you to revisit the question we started with and blank, hoping you will now conceive that your sharpest brain age is not in the past, but now or yet to come.

I was/am/will be sharpest at age _____.

In the next chapter, you will learn how to get a good vantage point into the health of your brain and become aware of how to strengthen your frontal lobe function, harness your brainpower, and increase your mental productivity while reducing preventable brain fatigue and losses at the same time. You will see how to take a good look at the condition of your own brain. You accumulate large savings in your brain account from preventive actions if you commit to building stronger brainpower. Challenge your brain's frontal lobe capacity. If you do, you will help to extend your brain span to more closely match your extended life span. Now that is a great gap to close.

Know Brainers

1. Your frontal lobe functionality powers your ability to thrive personally and professionally.
2. Frontal lobe fitness becomes increasingly more indispensable as you age.
3. Executive functions are more important for everyday life performance and independence than your IQ or intelligence quotient.
4. Your best brain years can be ahead of you, if you challenge your brain properly.
5. High-performance brain training can increase frontal lobe power.
6. You can build cognitive reserves that will add years to your brain's life and help build intellectual capacity in injury or disease.
7. Frontal lobe fitness rules, no matter your generation, no matter your life's work.

CHAPTER 3

A CHECKUP FROM YOUR NECK UP

Is cognitive decline inevitable? If so, when does it begin?
What are the essential cognitive brain capacities to benchmark and monitor?
Why get a brain benchmark when you are not worried about how your brain is working?
What age is prime for getting the first brain health benchmark?
How can intellectual capital (cognitive reserves) be built and stored?
Why is enhancing your brain edge a process rather than a product?

Each year you most likely have an annual checkup with your family practice physician or internal medicine doctor. Weight is noted, blood pressure taken, and cholesterol checked. All routine measures to keep your physical body in tip-top shape. The appointment is brief, and your doctor reminds you to exercise and eat right before sending you on your way. This annual routine establishes a benchmark of your physical health, one by which the next year's visit will be measured. What is not taken into consideration is your brain health, otherwise known as your cognitive fitness level.

> As life expectancy increases, so does risk for cognitive decline.

The Centers for Disease Control and Prevention reports the estimated life expectancy for this decade is seventy-eight. As I mentioned earlier, a health-care policy journal predicts that a mere forty years from now the average American life span for a man will be eighty-six years and for a woman ninety-three years.[1] Increased life expectancies pose numerous questions regarding what tips the scale from cognitive wellness into epochs of cognitive vulnerability. Think about these questions:

- What separates cognitive wellness from cognitive decline?
- Is cognitive loss a condition we will realize is transpiring or are the losses so insidious that they will be under our radar?
- When is cognitive slippage a concern and when is it just a momentary glitch of insignificance?
- Is it possible to stave off decline?

I often say, "Without brain health, we do not have health." The brain is the most vital organ to everyday-life functioning, and it is just as essential to measure and monitor your brain fitness as it is to measure and monitor your physical fitness. Being proactive is key to building healthier cognitive function, and significantly more needs to be done to achieve a brain health span that more closely aligns with our body's new life span. The potential to increase the number of years you have with maximum brainpower is here and now. Take advantage of it.

The majority of the population thinks that only a tiny window of time and opportunity is available to focus on and encourage optimal brain development. In fact, we focus almost exclusively on early childhood in terms of brain health development. This, of course, is a crucial life stage. However, it is too narrow a focus. Just as we have learned about the lifelong need to stay physically fit, **brain fitness requires lifelong efforts.**

> Create the foundation for prime brain function and build cognitive reserves.

A Benchmark for Brain Health

Six important discoveries about the brain are making us increasingly aware of the importance of keeping our brain in good operating function.

1. Our brain continues to make new cells every day we live.
2. The brain can form complex connections throughout life.
3. The connections between neurons can be strengthened against weakness.[2]
4. There is no time limit to brain repair. Previously, it was believed that the window for brain recovery was at most one year after injury; my research has shown that the brain can be repaired months and years after injury if higher-level demands are placed on frontal lobe skills.[3]
5. Restorative brain training practices share commonalities across diseases, injuries, and age related declines.[4–5] For example, thinking beyond the surface-level meaning of information can help build new or strengthen old connections after traumatic brain injury, stroke, in normal aging, and even in a progressive brain disease such as Alzheimer's.
6. Advances in sophisticated brain imaging technology allow us to view changes in the activation of brain regions that occur over the very moments we acquire new knowledge.[6] The changes in brain regions suggest there is more activation during learning. Brain regions work harder (thus requiring more glucose) when acquiring a new skill. As one begins to master the skill, these same brain regions show less activation because the brain does not have to work so hard to carry out the same heavy mental load.

I predict that preventive medicine will put brain health benchmark evaluations at the top of the list of best practices very soon. A brain health benchmark establishes a cognitive index of brain performance to determine current level of function and identify strengths and weaknesses. It allows you to monitor changes in your cognitive function and keep tabs on the stability or fragility of your cognitive fitness as you age. There is also a proactive element to having a benchmark, since it allows you to strengthen areas of weakness and continue to build resilience to guard against cognitive decline. In short, a cognitive assessment will help you better understand how your brain works, what it needs to be more fit, and ideas about how to achieve higher brain performance.

> A benchmark is needed to identify baseline performance as a metric to maintain cognitive brain health.

Presently, no simple test exists that has widespread acceptability to provide a benchmark of brain health. In fact, a simple assessment is not what we should be seeking; a *simple* test will never be sensitive or informative enough to index early failings in the complexities of our brain's capacity. An out-of-state group of talented doctors, who deliver an exceptional two-day comprehensive annual assessment of the body's overall health, came to me asking for advice in adding a brain evaluation component to their protocol. They said they needed something that would take no longer than thirty minutes because the checkup was already too long and cumbersome. I said, "Fortunately for each of us, the complexity of our brains does not lend itself to a simple thirty-minute assessment."

The Known versus the Unknown

> Fear is the greatest culprit to maintaining and strengthening brain health.

Fear of Alzheimer's disease keeps the majority of people in a perpetual state of dread and anxiety about seeking information regarding their brain status. However, when it comes to other health matters, we are often quick to act: checking our cholesterol for fear of heart attacks, watching our diet and exercising to maintain optimal physical health, avoiding sugars and high fat foods to prevent type 2 diabetes. When it comes to matters of physical health, **the known provides the necessary impetus to establish life-saving habits.**

In my research with returning war veterans, one Navy SEAL said, "We spend time doing everything possible to keep our bodies in the highest level of fitness. We would do anything to increase our body's performance edge. As I hear you talk, I am stunned that we have ignored the brain so much in our high-performance training. I want to be the first to get a brain health benchmark. I want to know what can be done to increase my clarity of thinking." And another Navy SEAL said, "Brain performance is the last frontier of human performance. How can we claim to be elite performers if we don't put the focus on the brain?" You, too, can make your brain health a known.

Establishing a brain benchmark is critical. If weaknesses are identified, there are proactive steps to regain cognitive ground. Doing so will strengthen these cognitive frailties early and support independent thinking for vital life decisions for years to come. Unfortunately, the knowledge that something can be done to improve brain health is not widely known. People still believe that if they get bad news about their brain, it is just that—bad news without hope.

> Increasing brainpower can elevate performance and lead to higher return in brainomics.

As you become a brain health advocate, you can become part of the movement to change this outdated and wrong information. **Brain science is revealing there are many ways to fight against brain decline.**[7-14] Optimal cognitive health is a desirable goal, since healthy brain function will be the greatest boon to our personal lives and our national productivity across the life span. But the first step is having a benchmark by which to measure improvement or decline. My team sees individuals for brain health benchmarks with so many different perspectives: (1) those who are excited to know as much as possible about their brain, (2) those who are anxious and do not really want to know, and (3) those who have benefited from establishing a benchmark before brain injury or brain disease.

Like many of the people who visit me, sixty-three-year-old John first made an appointment for a brain health benchmark because he was having memory troubles. Since memory is the most tangible part of the brain, it is this common struggle that lights the fire under individuals to check in on their brain's health. John confessed that his concern stemmed from a history of Alzheimer's disease in his family. Upon assessment, John demonstrated robust cognitive function, innovation capabilities, and creative insight into complex issues. He did struggle with detailed information and strategic attention, saying, "I'm a big-picture guy."

To address his minor weaknesses, my team recommended that he continue to capitalize on his ability to recognize the important ideas. He was then advised to write down specific details that were critical to remember, so he was not constantly worrying whether he would remember those particular facts or not, which could serve to overload his mental workspace and contribute to mental fatigue. He should not be trying to keep track of such information in his working memory space when he could refer to it where he wrote it down. We also encouraged him to assimilate and synthesize new ideas into bigger concepts based on the significant input to which he was exposed in meetings, from substantive emails, or from lengthy documents he had to read. Extracting meaning from complex data is one of the best ways to strengthen frontal lobe connections.

John wrote me after his assessment and follow-up, saying, "I feel invigorated and armed with the knowledge I need to 'mind the gap' and ramp up my brainpower." He commented that due to his family history of Alzheimer's, every time he forgot something, his fear and anxiety would skyrocket. He felt his worry was making his wife very concerned. He was beating himself up about letting so many details fall through the cracks that he was missing the mark on maintaining and even continuing to challenge his innovative thinking capacity. John was relieved when he learned that he did have memory problems, but the cognitive capacities that matter more were intact. He was now able to distinguish between what was a real worry versus what was a vulnerability. Armed with the tools to compensating for his vulnerabilities, John regained his intellectual confidence. He thanked my team for the enlightening, positive experience and said his only regret was that he had waited for so long in a worried state of mind.

And then there's fifty-nine-year-old Mary, a successful CEO, who did not seem to be tuned in to her cognitive slippage. It was not clear whether she was in denial or truly not cognizant of the changes that others could see. Mary was strongly encouraged to establish a brain health benchmark by a colleague who had observed some worrisome loss in her day-to-day performance. When she reported for her brain health checkup, Mary seemed unaware and oblivious to any problems and did not report any concerns about her brain function and current thinking capacity. However, she did

41

report that she often had difficulty remembering people's names and recalling information associated with them—though nothing unusual or worse than any of her friends.

Unconcerned as she completed the assessment, Mary put forth good effort on each cognitive task, but she struggled on every one. She demonstrated significant difficulty on all three key domains of frontal lobe functions (strategic attention, integrated reasoning, and innovation). She exhibited problems in blocking irrelevant data, synthesizing information, and remembering key ideas. Despite this overall low performance, Mary remained unmindful of her cognitive losses and to date has not heeded any of my team's recommendations. Since this was Mary's first brain health assessment, it was unclear how much slippage had occurred, but due to her level of achievement, clearly significant change had taken its toll on her brain's capacity.

Without insight, individuals may not make the necessary changes to take healthy steps to slow cognitive decline—just like with any health concern, whether it be diabetes and sugar or obesity and dieting. When I see clients like this, it causes me to work harder to increase public awareness before it's too late and too much loss has been incurred. What if Mary could have strengthened her cognitive functions earlier? Is it too late to ramp up Mary's cognitive capacity now? It's hard to know for sure and most likely some gains can be made, but one trend I do see is that when people lack insight into their problems, they rarely put in the effort required to make a difference. Sometimes lack of insight is a problem with frontal lobe function. Remember Phineas Gage in chapter 2, who was unaware of his deficits as a result of his brain injury? Change in insight capacity can also signal early signs of progressive brain concerns.

As we think about our brain's future, we need to adopt a comprehensive approach to brain health that is more thorough, more informative, more accurate, and more sensitive to establish a benchmark of brain health. You can join my movement to inspire your circle of influence to actively promote their cognitive brain's health. Everyone you inspire will be the biggest beneficiary.

Brain scientists have been working tirelessly to explore and discover the most sensitive and consequential measures of cognitive decline indicative of progressive brain diseases. Many of the widespread screenings are too low-level and superficial, asking questions such as:

- What day of the week is it?
- What season are we in?
- Who is the president? The vice president?

When you have problems with these questions, almost everyone knows, including the person questioned, that they have crossed the threshold from normal to disease. What if you were asked questions such as these?

- Explain what this saying means and apply it to a real-life circumstance: The long way home is often the fastest.
- Tell me about a complex project you recently completed and what actions you would change if you had it to do over and what you would do exactly the same. What are two things you added that have never been done before?
- Give me three specific ways you would improve health-care coverage and weigh how those changes would impact costs.

Leading-edge scientific teams have contributed significantly to our understanding of early symptoms of dementia and have focused largely on establishing measures to predict and detect Alzheimer's disease. What they have found is that cognitive measures are more sensitive than brain imaging or cerebrospinal fluid markers in predicting who would be most likely to develop Alzheimer's disease,[15-18] at least for now. My goal is not to focus solely on the brain in a state of injury or disease, but to apply the findings we have learned from these discoveries to healthy aging individuals like you to delay decline to the greatest degree and longest time period possible.

Utilizing complex cognitive measures and sophisticated brain imaging, my team and I have developed and tested measures to index the brain's strengths as well as areas that can be improved. Our cognitive assessment is called the BrainHealth Physical. Performance results are used to guide individuals on how to:

- Increase productivity
- Decrease brain fatigue
- Achieve higher levels of work efficiency
- Identify weaknesses in strategic attention
- Focus and stay on task

- Increase flexibility in thinking
- Be aware of habits that drain the brain
- Identify areas of strong mental reserve
- Recognize ways to strengthen core areas of vulnerability
- Increase brain energy

The BrainHealth Physical is a unique assessment of cognitive fitness that examines vital higher-order thinking abilities, such as strategic attention, integrated reasoning, innovative thinking, and mental flexibility. It is not an IQ measurement. It is not a brain scan. It is a mental stress test that measures cognitive abilities that can be enhanced and should remain robust as we age in the absence of progressive brain disease.

> Wouldn't you like to know what drains your brain's energy and regain energy instead of feeling brain exhaustion each and every day?

Clients are comforted by the amount of insight gleaned from their BrainHealth Physical. Jerry Hoag, the executive director of The University of Texas at Dallas School of Management Leadership Center, partnered with BrainHealth and offered BrainHealth Physicals to managers of the world's top corporations to give them an advantage on how to improve their leadership by understanding how to strengthen their own brain capacity. Mr. Hoag said, "So many tests administered to business executives do not inform them as to how to change their behavior."

After taking the BrainHealth Physical, the managers were given exercises to help them improve in areas that are vulnerable. The individual experienced what impacts his or her own brain health first. Then they learned how their leadership style could be either building or robbing their teams' highest brain performance.

We take better care of our cars than our brains by getting regular tune-ups. It is false to assume that the majority of individuals will no longer be able to make their own decisions due to a relentless loss of cognitive function. You can alter this downward course of events if you implement brain health practices now. Take the challenge to maintain and show gains in brain vibrancy in your core frontal lobe functions. Knowing where you stand now is the first step to building cognitive resilience.

> Robust brain health **does not** equal high IQ.

There are three main areas of informative metrics to monitor as we age in order to maintain robust cognitive function. You will learn more about each in the following three chapters. These include:

1. **Strategic Attention**—How proficient are you at strategically evaluating information? How efficiently do you decide what information is important to know versus what information should be ignored? Blocking information and avoiding distractions have become increasingly more difficult and a weakened cognitive skill in this day of information overload. How can we tell? Twenty- to thirty-year-olds, whom I refer to as the Finders, are the lowest performers of practicing strategic attention. The frontal lobe skills involved in strategic attention are pivotal as they are some of the leading predictors of a high-performing brain.

   Check out your strategic attention:

   - Can you walk/jog outdoors without music or other input through earphones?
   - Can you hold off for one-hour intervals to check email or phone messages?
   - How many people do you interact with during the day where you are "present" in the conversation without distractions—either doing another task or attending to thoughts in your head? Track the times it occurs—it is rare.

2. **Integrated Reasoning**—What is the status of your current capacity to apply new information across situations? How often do you absorb new content and quickly synthesize the meanings for a vast richness of generalized applications? To succeed in a competitive work environment, one must have knowledge of facts and an ability

to appropriately apply ideas and content at a more global context to strategically direct key changes in course and actions, and an ability to dynamically switch between the two. Switching, or quickly shifting focus between details at hand to bigger issues, is essential to successful brain function whether in the workplace, service of others, or home environments. Believe it or not, those older than sixty-five are best at this skill—despite our current belief that we are the most cognitively robust in our twenties.

Check out your integrated reasoning skills:

- How often do you finish an important phone call and synthesize your viewpoint and ways it converged and diverged from the person you were speaking with?
- Do you prepare bold challenge statements to kick off conversations—even at routine gatherings?
- Do you create subject lines that entice others to read your emails?

3. **Innovation**—How strong is your ability to engage in novel thinking? How ingenious are you at identifying and generating multiple innovative solutions to a problem by seeing different options and appreciating others' perspectives, especially those that differ from yours? Innovation requires novel thinking at every age and involves being nimble in our thinking, keeping our ideas fluid, and staying creative when it comes to problem solving. The Thinkers, or baby boomers, are on top of the pyramid in this skill, at present. But every generation can ramp up their creativity and innovation skills. I will tell you different ways to do so, but you have to first start by understanding that you have untapped potential to be more creative.

Check out your innovative thinking skills:

- How often do you go to the same restaurant and order the same food?

- How often do you pick up and read periodicals or sections of the newspaper you have never read before?
- When someone disagrees with your point of view, how often do you find a few reasons why he may have a differing but sound experience base?
- Do you do something novel each day?

Why do these three areas—strategic attention, integrated reasoning, and innovation—matter so much? These cognitive areas are the foundation to achieve brain efficiency, ensure mental productivity, and maximize brainpower. **These brain processes are the key ingredients for robust brain function and independence late in life.**

> "Vulnerable to aging" is a warning to do something, not a pessimistic edict proclaiming the unstoppable and inevitable.

As you learned in the last chapter, research shows that frontal lobe functions, in general, and reasoning, in particular, are vulnerable to aging.

This progression of cognitive vulnerability has naturally unfolded in many older adults who have not had the benefit of focused attention to improve their brain health. It is time to change the course for each of us. The good news is that you can.

To think about your brain health, you must go beyond the two cognitive skills that we often hold in highest esteem—speed and vast memory capacity.

1. **Speed:** How quickly do you complete a task such as completing a crossword puzzle, finishing a report, preparing a presentation, or cleaning out a closet?
2. **Vast memory capacity:** How would you rate yourself at remembering facts, such as all the medication and various doses you are taking, the major turning points of the Cold War, the names of all the people at an event recently, the names of your high school teachers, the capitals of all the states, or the elements in the periodic table?

We put too much value on speed and memory. Remember, speed of responding and vast memory capacity does not equate to best outcome, nor do they correspond to high brain performance. Early in my research career, I learned that these two prized cognitive assets might not be the pinnacles of brainpower that we all seemed to hold dear. I continue to see this lesson reinforced. In my first aging grant funded by the National Institute of

> Speed and quantity do not determine peak brain health.

Aging almost twenty-five years ago, I adopted the pervasive view that advanced aging and early dementia were not distinct entities but rather on a continuum, a perspective that is still widely espoused today.

That is, I hypothesized that adults between eighty and ninety-five would overlap considerably with younger adults (sixties and seventies) with early stage Alzheimer's disease. As often happens in scientific studies, my results were not at all what I expected. Yes, memory and speed of thinking in the cognitive healthy old-old adults, eighty to ninety-five years of age, were significantly lower; similarly, individuals with early-stage Alzheimer's disease in their sixties and seventies showed significant decline in these two areas. What I had not anticipated was that the old-old group were as cognitively capable as healthy adults in their sixties and seventies and even outperformed college students on measures of integrated reasoning and abstracting meanings. For example, when I asked my participants to interpret a long written text, older adults generated more responses and higher levels of generalized statements from a broader perspective than younger participants. To be quite honest, I was mildly shocked.

In contrast, individuals with very mild Alzheimer's disease were significantly impaired in the ability to convey abstracted meanings from complex content. Numerous studies have continued to reveal that higher-order synthesis of complex information is a vital cognitive skill that can be preserved, if not elevated to new heights, in healthy brain aging.[19–21]

Test yourself:

- Interpret as many meanings as you can from your favorite song lyrics.
- Practice devising a newspaper-

> Age is not an accurate predictor of decline in integrative thinking.

like heading to capture the essence of what you experienced during an evening out.

The key is to constantly push your cognitive performance to construct something novel and abstract. By doing so, you will begin to feel your brain energized and ramp up your brainpower.

Imagine the fifty- and sixty-year-olds and sixty-five-and-up participants outperforming the thirtysomethings at the cognitive skill of integrated reasoning. I would wager that the gap is widening each year. Today the young Finders (twenty- and thirty-year-olds) may be starting off at a weaker point when compared to other generations. Whereas Finders may be the strongest in areas of speed and quick recall of more facts, they do not have the accumulated experience and knowledge base to lead in integrated reasoning. Part of the problem is likely due to growing concern that the Finders are reading approximately 60 percent less than the Thinkers (fifties and sixties) generation. On the other hand, Finders may be taking in as much information—perhaps even more—just through different channels. Cognitive brain health depends not on how much information a person takes in but rather how deep the person is reinterpreting and creating new meaning from information.

Findings from my BrainHealth research team have shown that we can change the conversation of doom and gloom to one of hope and cognitive gain at each stage of life. **What's more, we can improve brain function in core areas that matter in the young and the old. But it all starts with awareness and benchmarking.**

Ask yourself these questions:

- How strategic are you in blocking extraneous input? How often do you make your brain do work in a noisy environment, when you could be working in a quieter context?
- How often are you reflecting on how to rethink a project—even when you cannot redo it?
- How often are you figuring out new ways to do things?

Just as the 1960s aerobic exercise movement got our bodies moving, efforts to motivate the public to get our brains in gear will have major payouts. We need to engage the frontal lobe in cognitively challenging activities that involve higher-order reasoning to strengthen and preserve cognitive capacity—regardless of age.

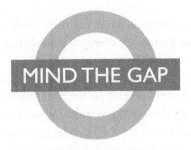

MIND THE GAP

"Mind the gap" is a warning that was coined in London in the late 1960s to warn Tube (or, underground) passengers of the potential danger in the gap between the station platform and the train door. Metaphorically speaking, nearly all of us possess brain gaps, or areas of cognitive function that are not performing to their optimal potential. If we do not mind our brain gaps continually every single day, the expanse between our lifespan and brain health span will grow wider—an overall gap that becomes increasingly more difficult to close. Just as passengers riding London's underground tunnel system are reminded to mind the gap between the train and the platform, you too want to heed this warning in terms of your brain and its performance. Tend to your cognitive gaps every day to build the most robust brain possible.

Think of your brain as a bank; you need to build your cognitive reserves, much as you would contribute to a savings account. This allows you to guard against cognitive decline. **Cognitive reserves are how much cognitive capacity you have built up or saved at any point in time to counter brain pathology either due to disease, injury, or age-related losses.** Research has proposed that the more cognitive reserve you accrue over the years, the more likely you are to be able to functionally stave off decline and guard against brain loss in terms of mitigating degrees of impairment. This explains why higher levels of education seem to be consistently associated with more protective cognitive capacity. How much is in your brain bank to counter the effects of brain loss? It is never too early or too late to start making deposits to your brain bank. For example, how often do you hear a fascinating interview on public radio or a talk show and share the meaningful messages you gleaned that are unique to you? To build reserves, you want to keep stretching your mind to extract big principles, not try to be a scribe of someone else's ideas. Stretch yourself to take on new mental challenges you have a natural affinity toward.

> Avoid challenges that drain your passion.

Though a real phenomenon, cognitive reserves are currently more of a theoretical construct than one that can actually be indexed. The term was conceived to help explain why people vary greatly in terms of the relationship between the degrees of brain damage and cognitive loss. For example, the same degree of Alzheimer's pathology may produce little cognitive impairment in one person and produce major cognitive impairment in another person. Similarly, my research in traumatic brain injury measured individuals with minimal brain damage who showed major cognitive problems as well as the reverse pattern.[22-25] That is, I evaluated those with severe brain damage who were able to recover high levels of cognitive functionality. So why is it that some brains experience minimal damage with major consequences? Whereas others suffer major injuries, and within months they are back to high functionality? Both may have similar pre-injury IQ but different cognitive reserves.

The lack of reliable correspondence between brain damage and cognitive performance has prompted researchers to explore this concept of cognitive reserves. Cognitive reserves mitigate the amount of brain loss that has to occur before evidence of cognitive impairment is manifested on measures or subjectively recognized by significant others in a person's life.[26-27]

The more cognitive reserves you have built up, the more protection you have for staving off decline resulting from the brain culprits that directly or indirectly damage the brain, e.g., chemotherapy, chronic stress, brain injury, stroke, or forms of dementia. When a person has lower levels of cognitive reserves stored, their cognitive capacity will likely be vulnerable to even small degrees of brain insult. In contrast, with higher reserve levels, the symptoms will appear later and be milder as compared to those with low

> Keeping your mind mentally active makes your brain's neurons healthier, longer.

reserves and similar degrees of brain insult. How do you build up cognitive reserves? By constantly engaging in complex mental activity.

You must decide today if you want to give your brain the best chance to rebound from injury or other brainpower thieves to be the strongest possible each day. You cannot wait a day to start actively working your brain. In fact, researchers find that people who are more cognitively active over their whole brain span have less amyloid buildup, an abnormal brain deposit associated with Alzheimer's disease.[28-30] If people wait to get their brain charged on challenges, the gains are less robust. Do you want to let your brain go backward? For the majority of people that is exactly what is happening.

Thus the higher levels of cognitive reserve you possess and build,

1. the longer you will be able to stave off cognitive decline.
2. the less severe the cognitive decline will be.

My research efforts over the past decade have focused on identifying brain-training regimens that can lengthen optimal cognitive functioning in meaningful ways critical for everyday life functions.[31-38] My findings are adding to the healthy brain

> Your brain is your most important organ and deserves your attention.

evidence that fluid intelligence and higher-order thinking capacity can be improved into late life if we implement the ABCs of brain health.

- A = **Awareness** of personal brain performance—strengths and vulnerabilities
- B = **Benchmark** of cognitive brain function as the starting point of a cognitive fitness plan
- C = **Conditioning** to conscientiously engage in complex and personally motivating mental challenges that draw upon the vast frontal lobe networks.

As mentioned earlier, one of the most overlooked aspects of performance is our brains' health. One of my clients, Steve, commented that he had always prided himself in being able to keep up with all the demands that were handed to him. Not until his brain benchmark had Steve realized the high cost of the stress he was under and information overload on his brain performance. He was having memory problems, unable to keep a coherent train of thought, and slipping in terms of his previous innovative thinking. He was motivated to turn things around and regain his cognitive losses. With specific strategies in place, Steve was determined to change his brain habits and recapture his brainpower potential through conditioning and practice.

Know that your brain is one of the most modifiable parts of your whole body. As the most important aspect of your health, it should be delegated a prominent position front and center. It is up to you to either be a lackadaisical brain athlete or an elite Olympic-level performer. With a healthy brain, longevity will be a boon to society and to our economic bottom line. In the next chapters, you will learn the necessary steps to maintain your brain function and improve its health so that the brain you have at seventy-five or ninety-five is even more robust than it is today.

For additional tools and tips visit www.makeyourbrainsmarter.com.

Know Brainers

1. Without brain health, we do not have health.
2. Get a benchmark of your brain's fitness level as soon as possible to make sure you rebound and maintain your cognitive capacity as long as possible.
3. The complexity of our brain core processes requires a sophisticated measurement of fluid intellectual capacity.
4. Continual learning and education builds protective cognitive reserves.
5. A brain health benchmark is perhaps more important than a physical checkup because it is the first step toward maintaining and strengthening capacity.
6. Brain health habits are vital at all ages; each stage of life has different cognitive challenges and potentials.

SECTION II

MAXIMIZE YOUR COGNITIVE PERFORMANCE

CHAPTER 4

STRENGTHEN YOUR STRATEGIC BRAIN HABITS

How strategic is your thinking?
What is the upside and downside of multitasking?
Are you a gatekeeper or do you crave data downloading?
Why is access to more information not making us smarter?
Learn how improving your brain health can be as simple as
remembering none, one, and two.
> *Brainpower of None*
> *Brainpower of One*
> *Brainpower of Two*
How can you take advantage of silence to increase your insightful
problem-solving capacity?
How can you advance your strategic task prioritization?

Your brain contains more than 10 billion neurons with more than 10 trillion connections, or synapses. The numbers are staggering, representing the most amazing and complex network imaginable. Your genetic makeup plays a key role as the architect of this intricate labyrinth; your brain, in general, and your frontal lobe, in particular, support unparalleled computational thinking, which, to be quite honest, no computer can come close to matching.

A thirty-five-year-old male client of mine announced to me, "More, more, more—the more I have access to helps me make better decisions." Joe, a highly successful professional who is actively involved in the community, attends every single meeting in and outside his office or town, seeks and keeps massive amounts of data constantly, and acts as the primary contact for many projects. He does not prioritize. He mistakenly thinks that **more is better.**

When asked if he had any concerns about his brain performance, he confessed, "My kids think I have a memory problem." Halfway joking and halfway not, he conceded, "I am having a little trouble. I feel like my brain is fried at the end of long days. I can't even keep their names straight, and I only have two kids!"

After our conversation, I assessed that his problem was not his memory. Joe, like many other high-achieving individuals, was pressing his brain to take in and manage as much as possible. Unfortunately, his relentless pace and info-craving habits were zapping his brain energy.

What is a strategic brain? When you use your brain strategically, it filters information by deliberately sorting input and output. The approach is two-pronged: (1) attending to necessarily essential information while (2) filtering out extraneous data that is less critical to the task at hand. In contrast, a nonstrategic brain takes in all information.

Despite the brain's immense processing capacity, it cannot take in every piece of input—it does have its limitations. Our brain is built to work dynamically and efficiently; by design, it is smart. It is not built to be a massive information storage processor. We need to stop and ask ourselves if we want to use up our brain's limited resource capacity by focusing on trivial and poorly vetted information. **Which type of brain are you building? A strategic or nonstrategic brain?**

Even if our brains could store and process endless amounts of information, you would not want to sort through it all. I am reminded of how Sherlock Holmes describes himself to Watson in *A Study in Scarlet.*

You see, I consider that a man's brain originally is like a little empty attic, and you have to stock it with such furniture as you choose. A fool takes in all the lumber of every sort that he comes across, so that the knowledge which might be useful to him gets crowded out, or at best is jumbled up with a lot of other things so that he has a difficulty in laying his hands upon it. Now the skillful workman is very careful indeed as to what he takes into his brain attic. He will have nothing but the tools which may help him in doing his work, but of these he has a large assortment, and all in the most perfect order. It is a mistake to think that that little room has elastic walls and can distend to any extent. Depend upon it, there comes a time when for every addition of knowledge you forget something that you knew before. It is of the highest importance, therefore, not to have useless facts elbowing out the useful ones.

Boost your brainpower: What are some take-home messages from this passage about Sherlock? By thinking about these, you will boost your brainpower.

For me, one thing is clear: you need to be selective and keenly strategic in terms of what you store in your brain's attic. Of course, knowing at the point of entry whether a piece of information will be useful is not always possible, but you definitely need an effective triaging system than most currently employ.

Do you ever stop at the end of a day to reflect on all the impressive feats your brain helped you achieve? You should. With seemingly little effort, the brain typically responds and carries out the many demands you constantly make of it. Therefore, it is often taken for granted. Instead of marveling at its magnificence, individuals tend to remember the glitches more often than not. Everyone thinks back on that day when they could not recall an individual's name, or walked into a room and forgot what they were there for, or the time when they had a brilliant idea or question but lost it when it was their turn to speak.

The immense power of your brains' intricate cognitive capacity is so much more sophisticated than a memory system. Still, people place an extraordinary value on memory. In a survey of five hundred adults, I asked for the number one thing they wish they could improve about their brainpower. More than 80 percent said they would wish for a better memory, even a perfect memory, if that could be achieved.

> The wish for perfect memory may be more of a curse than a blessing, if granted.

When a wish becomes reality, it may not be what you truly want at all. King Midas wished that everything he touched would turn to gold. His wish was granted, and he was exuberant until he touched his beloved daughter, who turned into a gold statue. If you were granted a perfect memory, it may be your greatest stumbling block in terms of brain health and higher-level thinking.

Your brain is updated moment by moment and hour by hour. In essence, you frequently get a new processing system. **Indeed, you have the potential to change your brain with everything you do that has some level of challenge, novelty, or variety.** My research has found an interesting paradox: when one focuses on remembering the minute details, it may adversely affect the ability to engage in more strategic abstract thinking.[1-2] In essence, trying to remember as many details as possible can actually work against being selective about what you let into your brain's attic. This pattern helps explain why access to more information is not, on its own, making us smarter. More likely, quite the opposite is true. Exposure to large volumes of information steals and freezes your brainpower. However, my research has also shown that when focused and engaged more in strategic, abstract thinking, it becomes easier to remember the details.

> Everything is a trade-off. The more you focus on details, the more difficult it is to decipher big ideas to take into your brain bank.

> Strive to build a strategic brain; a strategic brain is a brain changer and life changer.

Adults are pushing their brains so

hard to solve and complete more tasks than ever before. Produce, produce, produce is a familiar refrain heard in our own thoughts, in school, in the workplace, and at home. But to build a healthy brain, you must stop your brain drinking from a fire hose that is spewing vast amounts of information. What you need to dedicate yourself to is building a strategic brain.

For Linda, a high-level executive at a Fortune 500 company, interruptions are her biggest hurdles to overcome. "Interruptions, people stopping by my office, phone calls, and an exponentially increasing number of emails—each with a new response expected instantly—are robbing me of my productivity. I often leave the office feeling like I can never catch up no matter how hard or how long I work."

Yes, being and feeling overworked is a prevailing hazard of the workplace. My BrainHealth team trained Linda in specific ways to take back control and harness the full frontal capacity of her brainpower. Retaking control requires daily prioritization of one or two predominant tasks, rather than jumping back and forth from one distraction to another. Task jumping is an all too common practice that is failing to advance the most crucial tasks and hinders strategic working and deeper thinking. Read on to see how Linda changed her beliefs and habits about what being mentally productive means.

One of the biggest obstacles to brain health is that our belief system about productivity is inaccurate. We all too often measure our productivity by how quickly we respond to emails and phone calls, juggle countless demands each day, and cross off item after item on our long to-do lists. The problem is, most tasks are done quickly without thoughtful processing—and instead almost with mind-numbing automaticity. Our quick responses make us feel like we are moving forward at the speed of light—as if we are keeping our daily bicycle moving forward. But are we running over pieces of glass or nails that may flatten our tires into mental exhaustion, making us lose our brain balance?

For some, there is a sense of guilt when they don't respond immediately to interruptions.

I remember when a client of mine, Paul, asked me: "What if it's your boss who is demanding immediate responses? If I fail to be timely, I will not

> Openness to distractions is keeping your brain off balance.

be looked upon favorably. It's easy for you to tell me to stall rather than respond quickly, but you better let my boss know or I'll be coming to you when I fail to get promoted."

I replied, "You are absolutely right. There must be buy-in at all levels—especially management. Leaders are some of the leading offenders—causing the state of constant distractedness and shooting themselves in the foot by reducing their team's productivity."

The guilt you feel from not responding instantly spurs you into action but does not pay off in terms of brain efficiency. For many, your competitive nature makes you your own worst enemy. We think we can do everything well, in record time, regardless of task.

Take Jim. A middle-level manager, he once told me, "I feel like I'm in a competition with myself and my team. It makes me feel worthy and important to know the answer and to be the first to send the answer out." But a polar opposite of Jim is Carmen, a woman I recently worked with who noticed the following: "I've found that if I don't respond immediately or engage in knee-jerk reactions, most of the problems solve themselves. Instead of a flurry of emails trying to solve a problem instantly, I let the problem take its course (if it's a nonemergency) and strategically select when to attend to it. By that time, eighty-five percent of the problems are solved and no response is necessary."

Dorie Clark, in a *Harvard Business Review* article titled "Five Things You Should Stop Doing in 2012," recommended that people stop responding to email like a "trained monkey."[3] She commented on how responding to email was becoming like a "slot machine for your brain"—with variable interval reinforcement. In fact, few of our emails require immediate responses. As Clark writes, "A 90-minute wait won't kill anyone, and will allow you to accomplish something substantive during your workday." I couldn't agree more.

Through my research, I've found that more than 87 percent of professionals report that they are interrupted more than 80 percent of their day, making it difficult to take even five minutes to deeply ponder the important work needed to be accomplished or thinking through ideas that would advance major conference calls concerning key problems. Much effort is wasted because we have not allowed space and time to ponder. **The unfiltered, massive influx of new information competing for your consideration and the constant interruptions from cell phones chirping, emails**

dinging, and in-person intrusions rob you of clear, strategic, insightful thinking. Constant interruptions are depleting your productivity. These interruptive expectations and environments are increasing rather than decreasing, causing a higher incidence of interruptions. The result is lower performance, more errors, and greater stress.

Rather than being strategic about how we use our brain time, we nurture and pride ourselves on how many emails and phone calls we receive and respond to each day. Rather than trying to fend off our addiction to being continuously available, we are reachable at all times, day or night, at work or at home. Until now, brain science had not discovered that such rapid exchanges of communication hinder rather than help your brain's competitive edge.

Nathan Zeldes, a former IT principal engineer at Intel Corporation and now principal at Nzeldes.com, wrote an article in 2007 titled "Infomania: Why We Can't Afford to Ignore It Any Longer."[4] Zeldes and his colleagues, David Sward and Sigal Louchheim, define "infomania" as the mental state where one is addicted to information downloading—an insatiable quest for additional information. This addictive habit is tough to break despite the continuous stress and distraction caused and, in essence, this infomania is detrimental to our brains.

> Our addiction is an insatiable craving for and an inability to be separated from technology. Our ability to constantly access more information may be the very thing that is contributing to our sickness.

Over time, your cognitive ability to focus and think deeply about one or two reputable information sources may be diminishing as a result of your habits. The brain's ability to inhibit how much information reaches its sphere of attention is weakening, meaning that the frontal lobe may become faulty, unreliable, even disrupted. In short, you may be reprogramming your brain to be exhausted, unfocused, and constantly responsive to interruptions. You are putting your intellectual capital at risk—daily.

"Each day I can feel my blood pressure rise as new information and

> A voracious addiction to information is toxic to your brain's productivity.

an influx of new action items from emails, meetings, and conversations are thrown my way," Linda, the Fortune 500 company executive, said before her BrainHealth Physical. "I force myself to absorb volumes of information."

Are you able to strategically attend to tasks at hand?

Ask yourself these questions to determine how vulnerable or how robust your strategic attention is:

- Do you allow frequent interruptions (three to four per hour) when you are working on your main tasks?
- Do you jump to a new task when immediately asked rather than making good progress on the major goal of the day?
- Do you multitask more than twice a day when you're working on a major project or work with background noise that your brain may actively have to block out?
- Do you work past your regular bedtime two nights or more a week to solve complex problems or complete major assignments?
- Do you have difficulty knowing when you have saturated your capacity to think clearly and work effectively?
- Do you recognize when there are strains on your task performance?

If you answer yes on two or more of these questions, your strategic attention requires an overhaul.

Whose fault is it that you remain in a constant state of distractibility? Is it due to your rapidly changing world, your boss, or yourself? **It seems adults today literally strive to be distracted, unable to allow a solo entry of input for even brief lengths of time.**

Microsoft researchers studying productivity taped twenty-nine hours of people working in a typical office, and found that they were interrupted on average four times each hour.[5] Additionally, 40 percent of the time, the person did not resume the task they'd been working on before the interruption. The more complex the task, the less likely the person was to resume working on it after an interruption.

Boost your brainpower: Track yourself. How often do you spend more than ten minutes on one task at home or at work?

In addition to being continuously ready for any distractions (email chirping, texting, pinging), if you are like many adults, you have a strong attraction and bias toward overstimulation and massive data downloading. The immense information downloading is taking an insidious toll on each of us, and yet we falsely believe we are thriving on infomania. And on a personal level, these consistent and ever-increasing interruptions are related to **elevated stress levels,** i.e., increased cortisol, frustration, more sickness, and hampered creativity.

Do you often feel your brain is extraordinarily fatigued at the end of the day? You may be failing to develop and strengthen strong frontal lobe strategies to hierarchically organize the information to which you must attend and the information you can throw out. It is like staring at the sun and being unable to see it because of the brightness. There is no way your mind can remember everything. Information overload is blinding your mind.

Strategic attention involves removing yourself from information absorption to solve problems. It is the ability to block and filter distractions while focusing on a central task. Focus is not just concentrating on the context at hand but, more important, it is about knowing when to step away and when to close off your mind from distractions. As Kenny Rogers would say, "You gotta know when to hold 'em, know when to fold 'em." That is exactly what we must do to improve our strategic attention:

> "Know when to hold 'em, know when to fold 'em."

know when and what to regard versus when and what to disregard.

Improving Strategic Attention

Your frontal lobe acts as your gatekeeper—letting in certain information while blocking out the rest. If you work hard to attend to as much information as possible, the brain gets overwhelmed and fails to reach its potential.

Science is revealing ways to maintain and strengthen your brainpower and improve your strategic attention, leading to increased productivity and overall well-being. **One key way to revolutionize the way you learn, energize your imagination, and ignite a deeper level of thinking is to be more strategic about how much information you take in at one time and how much effort you spend blocking out distracting information.**

> Strategic attention is based on the brain principle that less is more.

When you improve your strategic attention, you will develop habits to take back control of your time versus being controlled by your to-do list. You can take advantage of the vast potential of frontal lobe networks by sculpting your strategic attention habits.

Strive to develop and bolster strategies to enhance your strategic attention. How do you do it? You need to proactively and consciously establish core habits to prioritize goals and extract the goal-relevant ideas or features from the massive input you face.

Boost your brainpower: Practice strategically attending to a core task for a minimum of fifteen minutes at a time without interruptions.

With practice, the brain has amazing potential to filter out much of the superfluous information flooding our senses. But the problem is that we are engaging in hypervigilance—focusing on everything. Tony Schwartz, president and CEO of the Energy Project and author of *Be Excellent at Anything,* wrote an article for the *Harvard Business Review* on the importance of doing one thing at a time.[6] He warned that our major problem today is that we have lost our stopping points, finish lines, and boundaries. He warned that we are spending too many continuous hours juggling too many things at the same time. I agree. It has gotten so bad, we do not even believe we can do one thing at a time—nor do we want to. After reading this book, one of the biggest takeaways and easiest habits to implement is doing one thing at a time. Once you see how much more productive you are, you will not go back.

Track your own multitasking. For three days do the following:

- Chart the length of time per day you are able to focus on one and only one task without doing another single thing at the same time.
- Note how many tasks you work on longer than fifteen minutes without interruption.
- Note how many sidesteps arose because you were multitasking or allowing yourself to be pulled off task by distractions.
- Be aware that one of the major culprits to multitasking is the abundance of thoughts that fill your mind while you are doing something else.

We are forcing our minds to stretch their limited resources to actively ignore and simultaneously focus. As a result, we are doubly punished. This explains why clear thinking seems to be getting harder, regardless of age. But thinking doesn't have to be so arduous if you make just a few adjustments.

> Your brain has to work hard to ignore and filter information just as it works hard to focus on information.

We often work in cluttered, noisy environments that push our brains to put forth an inordinate amount of effort just to actively block information. No wonder many of us are overworking and fatiguing our brain! Now that you realize you are having to work extra hard to block out stimulation, will you rethink your environment?

Scientists are working hard to develop markers to show brain efficiency in selecting and inhibiting information. It's just as essential to block information that's unimportant and irrelevant as it is to selectively attend to necessary information. When

> In the near future, a brain biomarker could determine one's frontal lobe integrity by measuring the brain's capacity to inhibit and its ability to attend.

people say, "I wish I could improve my concentration and my ability to focus," I advise them it may be more productive to improve their ability to ignore—and then their ability to focus will be sharpened.

I have determined that there are at least four different profiles into which individuals can be categorized, determined by the characteristics of their strategic attention.

Strong Strategic Attention

1. **Strategic attenders:** Individuals who fall in this category learn over time and practice to employ strategies to improve their performance.
2. **Quick studies:** Quick-study performers adopt strategies immediately and continue to improve their performance as well as show generalized benefits to improving basic memory span.

Inefficient Strategic Attention

3. **Strategy-less:** These individuals try to remember everything without applying a strategy, failing to focus on particular information while ignoring other less relevant information.
4. **Faulty gatekeepers:** These individuals not only try to remember everything, but they also let the gates open too wide so that irrelevant information, even information that was never presented, intrudes on their learning and thinking.

What would your profile be?

Thirty-seven-year-old Doug does not practice gatekeeping. Even during his BrainHealth Physical, where he was asked to complete one task at a time, he was multitasking. Like many, Doug's chief multitasking distraction was taking place inside his own head. His internal thoughts were keeping him from being present. As a small business owner, Doug is involved in both strategy development and tactical execution at his company. However, his inability to attend strategically to important information while blocking out unimportant information is limiting his brain potential. No wonder he is struggling to move to a higher level of strategic planning.

Jane, a thirty-year-old communications professional, recently went through a BrainHealth Physical. She reported difficulty focusing on one task for an extended period of time, partly due to the nature of her job. With constantly changing circumstances and a pressure to respond to

> Stop blinding your mind. Step away and stop the flow and gluttony of information overload.

phone calls and emails quickly, she struggled to maintain strategic attention. In addition, Jane felt pressured to gather as much information as possible to form a well-grounded point of view to lead her clients down the correct path toward increased third-party credibility.

With a full explanation of strategic attention and recommendations to enhance the necessary cognitive process, she now practices ways to strategically attend to what is important and eliminate what is not. The result is a more efficient brain, increased creative thinking, and higher productivity. Specifically, Jane was given the following recommendations to reduce her brain fatigue:

1. Identify an issue/task each day for which she would like to find a better solution than the current practice and step away to take time to reflect on possible solutions. Within the week, offer her insights to her boss to show her independent and strategic thinking.

2. Practice interval training with email communications. Set regular times to attend to email and stop when time is up—for example, schedule twenty minutes three times a day. Only work on emails at that time—not simultaneously trying to do another task. The email messages will be more thoughtfully conveyed, standing out to recipients as being more thought-filled rather than reactionary. Do not spend your best brain hours deleting emails as it is a major time gobbler and gives a false sense of forward progress.

3. Reduce exposure to the amount of information she is being inundated with each day so that she can focus on one or two of the most important sources.

There are three strategies you can implement in your daily life to enhance your strategic attention. You will learn about these three core strategies below:

- **Brainpower of None**
- **Brainpower of One**
- **Brainpower of Two**

The Brainpower of None

How often do you work harder and harder to solve a problem? What if the brain solves problems best by taking a break from the matter? Have you ever noticed that when you struggle to solve a problem, you sometimes receive the answer just before you go to sleep or right when you wake up in the morning? Connections are built when brain activation slows, and even when our brain is at rest.

> Sleep is good for strategic thinking.

Brain scientists are beginning to show that when the mind quiets down and brain activity slows, we are able to connect the dots in new ways. When we are in a frenzy, frantically searching for answers, we do more to handicap our minds than to actually solve the problem; we are pushing our brains to the limits, failing to discover fresh insights.

Think back to when you could not remember the name of the person walking toward you; instantly you were embarrassed because you were well aware of all the facts about them, such as how you knew them, where they lived, and even their children's names. But your mind was frantically searching for that person's name, to no avail. Then somehow—out of the blue—

> Brain Paradox: Your brain works smarter when you make it slow down.

when you were no longer trying, perhaps on your drive home from the encounter or when you were brushing your teeth, the person's name came to you, clear as a bell. Why it could not come to your mind when you needed it demonstrates a glitch in the brain's search-and-rescue mission of immediately retrieving desired information that exists in your memory storage system. This simple example shows how you recall data when your mind is at rest.

Many report that they find themselves doing their best, most insightful thinking when they're half asleep, in the shower, or on an airplane—when they have been removed from their habitual hectic life context, precisely when they quit trying so hard. Now that is a mind marvel!

Solving problems or searching for an answer is not just about focusing and blocking distractions; it is also about stepping back to let the mind rest. Science suggests that a calm brain is more apt to trigger creative ideas and stimulate breakthrough thinking to solve complex problems when we hit a mental impasse. Joydeep Bhattacharya, a professor at Goldsmiths University of London, found that he could predict when people would solve insight puzzles based on their slowed EEG activity.[7] How? Steady alpha waves were seen on the right side of the brain, which is associated with a relaxed brain.

> Our brain works for us when we quit working it to the max.

Even more intriguing about how our brain works is that when participants in Bhattacharya's study showed strong gamma rhythms (as contrasted with alpha waves) after requesting clues to help solve problems, their brains seemed to be less open to using the clues to solve problems. Bhattacharya went on to suggest that when the brain is working hard to solve a problem, it basically froze the adults in their ability to benefit successfully from the additional clues they were given. Their minds seemed to get stuck and were not able to identify new options to solve the problem in front of them as opposed to being mentally nimble and flexible in seeing new possibilities. Although how alpha and gamma patterns predict brain states is still a bit controversial, brain scientists speculate that a relaxed brain allows the frontal brain regions to connect seemingly disparate and distant information to create novel solutions (see chapter 5 on integrated reasoning).

In his *New Yorker* article titled "The Eureka Hunt," Jonah Lehrer vividly described the real-life story of Wag Dodge, a man caught in the middle of a major fire in Montana while leading his team of fifteen firefighters to battle an out-of-control blaze in 1949.[8] Dodge saw the fire coming very close, and he did something very much against natural human instinct. He stopped. In that moment of pause, he had a flash of insight that saved his life. He lit a match that quickly set the slope around him on fire, then wet his kerchief and lay down amid the smoldering surrounding ground. Thirteen firefighters died trying to outrun the fire, but Dodge came away untouched. He could not explain how or where the idea came from, but in taking pause, a life-saving solution came to mind.

I refer to this as the **brainpower of none**. Big ideas often come when the brain stops frantically trying to solve the issue at hand. The brain thinks more clearly when it is seemingly doing nothing or is in a calmer state (since the brain is really never at rest—thank goodness!). We often experience major aha moments when we stop trying and clear our minds.[9] Often when we are practicing the brainpower of none, our brain's frontal lobe continues to search, change strategies, and start thinking in new ways.

> Searching for more information to make a decision? Stopping the search may make you smarter and more decisive!

Aha moments, or episodes of insight, are recognized as:

- A breakthrough after feeling like you were hitting a mental wall
- Seeing new ways to solve problems that did not seem to exist before
- Having a feeling of certainty that an idea will work
- Engaging in bigger-view thinking more than rationale thought

When we solve issues, we are often surprised we could not see the solution before. Does this mean you should not work hard to solve problems or complete tasks? Absolutely not! But you have to know when to practice the **brainpower of none**, giving your brain rest to allow new insights to emerge. Your frontal lobe works for you in creative ways when you step back.

> Use silence to think deeply, see things differently, and solve perplexing issues.

It is becoming increasingly rare to find times when people truly practice the brainpower of none. Instead, individuals constantly fill their thought-space with added stimulation. Take Patti, for example. She said her best downtime was when she was running. I said, "Terrific. Tell me about your running regime—do you observe nature or have music in your ears?" She said, "Oh, I definitely use an iPod with my favorite tunes when I run." I responded, "Having to actively block music from your mind, your brain is working rather than being freed up to make new connections. Therefore, running with an iPod is not downtime for the brain."

Others suggest driving in the car as their downtime. Again, many cannot stand the quiet. Try finding a time when your environment is truly quiet without any background stimulation to have to block out. When do you actively make time to have the **brainpower of none**? Incorporating time windows of silence in your hectic schedule will advance your complex thinking capacity.

Practice the **brainpower of none**, when you experience:

- Brain fatigue
- Information overload
- A major decision without clear direction
- A dead end to an issue
- Frustration and negativity

Boost your brainpower: Take time away and allow your brain to rest. To have your next aha moment, don't overthink it.

The Brainpower of One

Can you imagine a life without multi-tasking? With technological advances, we are readily able to do more; in other words, we are expected and addicted to doing more at once. Résumés from recent grads that come across my desk

Take your mind off your old thinking to discover a new way of thinking.

often include the words "efficient multitasker" or "ability to multitask" in a list of notable skills. With a constant connection to email, a cell phone, and the Internet, we have trained people to believe that multitasking is the key to success; we take pride in the ability of how much both others and ourselves can do at the same time.

Whenever I give a lecture on strategic attention and the **brainpower of one,** I often begin by raising my right hand and saying, "Hi, my name is Sandi, and I'm a recovering multitaskaholic."

It's true. I spent the first stage of my career juggling multiple tasks at the same time, thinking I was accomplishing everything at lightning speed and with the greatest efficiency. However, with more experience and knowledge of how the brain works, I learned that multitasking was one of the most toxic things I was doing to rob my brain of energy and high mental performance.

> Are you a multitaskaholic?

Yes, there are seemingly positive benefits to multitasking:

- Immediate access to massive amounts of information
- Greater input from multiple sources
- Ability to work faster
- Enhanced capacity to respond to more people in less time
- Being allowed to do more at the same time

But we have to stop and ask ourselves: What is our addiction to multitasking costing us? I asked myself this question years ago, and the answer I found changed my life forever.

Research has shown that if we counted all of the time we spend doing various tasks simultaneously, we'd actually be working an impossible forty-six-hour day and a 322-hour week, instead of our rampant 24/7.[10] No wonder we are so brain fatigued all day! Multitasking is bad for your brain and actually weakens your higher-order thinking capacity. Cognitive testing and brain imaging research reveals that multitasking causes

> Do you find yourself stretched to a breaking point? Do you often have trouble sleeping?

- shallower and less focused thinking;
- increased errors; and
- a dramatic negative decrease on mental processing.

Think about the impact of multitasking and frequent interruptions to task performance:

> Multitasking diminishes strategic attention.

- High mental productivity requires periods of single-minded tasking.
- The concept of doing one thing at a time is not being rewarded in the workplace, at home, by individuals, or by bosses.
- On average, we work for a total of only three minutes with laser focus, with no multitasking or interruptions.
- Once interrupted, it takes, on average, twenty minutes to return to the original task.
- In total, adding the time we are distracted and the time it takes us to return to the original critical task to complete it equals 2.1 hours! If only we could recoup all that time!

The lost time is not the only major cost. Multitasking actually makes us sick. It leads to a buildup of cortisol, the stress hormone that decreases our memory and contributes to increased brain cell death. Some scientists have even suggested that a buildup of stress and elevated cortisol levels is a major contributor to pathological conditions such as dementia.[11–13]

Our brain could have fooled most of us into thinking we are superior multitaskers! When asked, most people believe they are just as proficient when doing two things simultaneously. This is not true. We are wearing down our brains—literally fatiguing them with our constant demands to attempt two activities at the same time. The brain's frontal lobe has to quickly toggle back and forth while performing the two tasks. Your brain is built as a single channel action system with limited capacity; it bottlenecks when trying to do more than one thing at a time, except in very rare cases.

When you superimpose a second

> Simply put: your brain is not wired to do multiple things at once.

or even third task on top of doing something else, you saturate your mental capacity.[14] You are working your frontal connections harder to fight off interference from the flow of information. When pursuing a single goal, your frontal lobe works efficiently. When pursuing two goals concurrently, your frontal lobe power is divided and decreased.[15] If you add a third task to your attention dashboard, your errors increase dramatically, as much as tripling. This huge increase in errors reveals the severe limitation of our human cognition task overload. The debit to your intellectual capital is costly.

> What is on your brain's dashboard at this very moment?

People who are addicted to multitasking always want to challenge this finding. They say, "Maybe most people cannot, but I know I can multitask." And they are absolutely right. There are exceptions to the impossibilities of multitasking. When one or more of the tasks we are trying to complete are automatic (i.e., requiring less controlled thinking), it is possible to do two things precisely at the same time. For example, think of when you have folded laundry and held a conversation at the same time. Marcel Just and his colleagues at the Center for Cognitive Brain Imaging at Carnegie Mellon studied whether people could drive in a simulated driving task while having their brain scanned as they listened to spoken sentences and judged whether they were true or false.[16] The researchers were trying to mimic talking on the cell phone while driving, but admitted that judging sentences was not equivalent to deep conversation between the driver and the person on the other end, making it a more automatic task.

> Heavy multitaskers are building inefficient brains. Multitaskers have difficulty blocking out irrelevant input from their environment.

Nonetheless, in 2008 Just and colleagues still found a significant deterioration in driving accuracy (i.e., more driving errors) when research participants were processing sentences. Moreover, there was significantly less activation in the brain area (parietal lobes) devoted to the spatial processing necessary for driving ability—as much as a 37 percent reduction. The researchers suggested that their failure to find differences in frontal lobe activation as identified in other studies during multitasking might be due to more automaticity in both of their experimental tasks. For the brain, the task of processing sentences while simulating driving is not exactly comparable nor as challenging as dealing with all the life-threatening factors competing for our attention when driving in dense traffic on superhighways.

Now, all this is **NOT** to say that you should stick to one task for extended hours on end. **Your brain gets bored if fixed on one task too long.** Clearly, task toggling has its rewards. It helps to refresh one's mind. You may find that you are more mentally energized when you return to a complex task after a break to work on a separate issue. You just need to strike a balance between these two.

Boost your brainpower: instead of multitasking, perform tasks sequentially and remember the brainpower of one—focus on one task at a time, even if only short segments of time.

The Brainpower of Two

To-do lists are great and absolutely necessary so you're not forced to repeatedly remind yourself of the things you need to accomplish—a brain drain in itself. We have been trained to use to-do lists to organize our days. But, all too often, we have too many to-dos without any reflection of prioritization, leaving us feeling overwhelmed just by the sight of the list. They also fail to reflect a looming deadline and very often lack the necessary precision to tell us where to start and what to do here and now. Looking at an endless list of tasks freezes our minds.

More often than not, to-do lists consist of simple tasks to move the ball forward on a project such as the following: email so and so, call this person, check in with that person, or complete a specific document. If you're like most when looking at a massive to-do list, you choose to do the easiest things on the list, or tasks that can be completed in a measurable amount of time, so you can have the satisfaction of crossing something off the list. However, this process saves the difficult tasks that require more strategic thinking for later, when your brain is more tired. We are working and attending to distractions immediately and continually functioning well below our brain's potential. With the constant state of fragmented focus, our brainpower is kept at a very superficial level.

Remember Linda, the principal at a Fortune 500 company? After becoming more aware of her brain health and the importance of sequential tasking and not multitasking, she allowed herself the freedom to engage in continuous deep thinking on main tasks at certain time intervals. She intentionally assigned and gave the majority of her time to her highest priority and top-ranking tasks, investing wisely in her intellectual capital.

> To increase the return on investment in your intellectual capital, you need to focus on the highest priority task, and not invest time in a wide range of "junk" investments.

Linda explained the difference to me. "Professionally, improved strategic attention has helped me change how I allocate my time at work. I have forced myself to change my habits of instantaneous responding to most every interruption by practicing interval training with laser-focused blocks of work time. I no longer allow myself to be constantly interrupted, even by my own thoughts of the next small thing to do. Focusing on my major projects and not allowing time-gobbling constant disruptions has helped tremendously. I now set aside designated slots of time devoted to email and returning phone calls rather than being available all day long. I cannot believe the difference it has made to allow me to be more 'present' in each of the activities I'm involved with throughout the day."

> As T. Boone Pickens would say, "When you're hunting elephants, don't get distracted chasing rabbits."

She continued, "Becoming aware and doing something to strengthen my strategic attention relieved my stress by showing me that I really could take back control of my out of control schedule and still be highly productive and responsive."

Boost your brainpower: When you write your to-do list, focus on the two things—your elephants—that will have the most impact, require the most attention, the most rested brain effort and strategic thinking.

Don't get distracted chasing rabbits down endless trails all day long. Start using your copy of the elephants and rabbits **brainpower of two** to-do list at the end of this chapter. Identify your one or two elephants for the day—those are your top priorities. Be aware that rabbits should not turn into elephants; they truly are less important tasks.

Linda agrees with this approach. "Instead of constantly multitasking and crossing off less-essential items from my to-do list, I now concentrate on my pivotal goals for the majority of my working hours. When I need a break, I take care of some rabbits. I constantly reassess my schedule to make sure I am spending the largest chunk of my time tending to my elephants—the most important and vital tasks to being productive that day. I now realize if I neglect my elephants, they may run over me. Not so for my rabbits; they keep coming back. Learning about my brain health and how I was being inefficient with even the scheduling of my to-do list has had a major impact on my productivity and, in fact, has led to even stronger work output. I am even designing a sign to post on my closed door: 'Do not disturb—taking care of elephants!'"

To be mentally smarter, we must constantly reevaluate and identify one or two top priorities that demand the bulk of our energized brainpower, not the leftover, burned-out energy. Even in the midst of doing an activity, we should ask ourselves: "Is the task that is currently consuming my brainpower the activity that I need to devote my longest attention to because it will have the greatest impact?"

Boost your brainpower: Strategically attend to your two most important tasks every day.

To boost your cognitive function, you must harness the power of strategic attention and build a brain that filters and focuses. Doing so will increase your productivity and lead to improved well-being. Strategic attention alone is the most action-oriented step to maximizing your cognitive potential, but it cannot be done alone. Learn more about the important brain process of integrated reasoning in the next chapter.

Know Brainers

Brainpower of none: When you hit a mental wall, quiet your mind to regain brain energy and find fresh solutions. Learn to use silence to solve perplexing problems and think deeply.

Brainpower of one: Work on one thing at a time. Sequential-task instead of multitask. Secondly, strategically block a large percentage of incoming information and consciously know what to select.

Brainpower of two: Every day identify and dedicate the majority of time to your two most important "elephant" tasks.

Make Your Brain Smarter

_____

_____

_____

_____

_____

_____

_____

_____

_____

_____

_____

_____

makeyourbrainsmarter.com

CHAPTER 5

ENHANCE INTEGRATED REASONING TO ACCELERATE PERFORMANCE

How does complex mental activity rewire your brain to be healthier?

Why does continually engaging in integrated reasoning make your brain more efficient?

In what ways does engaging in complex mental activity, such as integrated reasoning, improve the biological health of the brain?

When and why should you transform incoming facts into abstracted ideas?

How do challenging integrated reasoning activities keep your fluid intelligence from going backward?

What activities and contexts provide rich opportunities to expand your integrated reasoning capacity?

How can the principles of integrated reasoning be exploited to energize meetings and inspire email communications?

What are ways to improve integrated reasoning capacity to accelerate strategic leadership skills?

Do you feel that those around you are able to:

• Express an idea you had been thinking, but say it with weighty impact and perfectly worded?

- Write emails that express ingenious thinking that garner positive traction?
- Interact on conference calls with comments that have lasting and strong influence?
- Generate promising solutions that others start immediately deliberating over?

Integrated reasoning is a rich, multifaceted, ubiquitous, and impressive mental capacity that, if regularly practiced, can revolutionize your brain health habits and your mental intellect.

You think you might have as much potential as any person does, but then you are not sure. Is it confidence? Is it social wherewithal? Or is it that such individuals have taken advantage of opportunities and expended the effort to be an entrepreneur of ideas? Have they developed regularly practiced habits of complex mental processing? I would wager the case is the latter. Remember the opening story of this book? We have long believed (the majority still believe) that we are either born smart or not. **Discard this outdated conventional wisdom today, this very minute. There is nothing you cannot get better at doing.**

Whereas it may seem that it comes naturally to others, well-formed innovative ideas are more typically the by-product of long-standing, effortful, dynamic thinking habits and content processing patterns. This mental habit can improve integrated reasoning levels regardless of age. Its expansion requires time and effort. To improve your skills in the bulleted points above, think deeply, and integrate those thoughts in your communications throughout your day. Even use silence to free the mind to imagine possibilities. Take the challenge to engage in complex mental activity daily by practicing integrated reasoning and you will advance your personal skills as a CEO, aka Cognitive Entrepreneur Officer.

Integrated reasoning is your brain's platinum cognitive asset. Really. Integrated reasoning is fundamental to all major goals you strive to achieve, decisions you make, projects you orchestrate, and major life changes and choices. This platinum asset requires continual fortification. On the upside, you can elevate your integrated reasoning capacity immediately. Do not be stuck and squelch your potential based on what others have told you at some point along your life path. You have immense potential to excel whatever your stage of life. On the other hand, if you perceive yourself as being relatively strong in integrated reasoning, cautiously remember that strong at one stage will not hold unless regularly practiced. Integrated reasoning is a skill that atrophies relatively quickly without practice.

Integrated reasoning is represented by these mental activities:

- Generating synthesized ideas
- Reconciling and updating novel ideas within the context of your rich knowledge base
- Extracting and altering broad principles from complex input
- Creating broader and new ways of thinking and acting
- Dynamically changing old practices by cultivating original thinking
- Reflecting on and discontinuing outdated old principles that are stifling entrepreneurial thinking

Integrated reasoning is transformative thinking. When you become astutely aware of the distinction between when you employ integrated reasoning habits of thinking versus insidious rote thinking patterns, you will see and experience a brain gain in a relatively short time period. Integrated reasoning is the fundamental principle for your brain's lasting resilience that ensures you do not lose ground. It is imperative to continue to exercise your integrated thinking muscle daily. See in the chart on page 85 some differences in integrated reasoning and insidious rote thinking on important tasks.

What does it mean to synthesize ideas: to construct novel, generalized thoughts? To synthesize meaning requires taking in facts, filtering the meanings, and transforming these into abstract concepts by drawing upon the rich experiences and knowledge that come from your uniquely built mind.

Activity	Integrated Reasoning	Rote Thinking
Meeting Planning	Set novel goals, write desired outcomes; have each attendee abstract their take-home message; determine next best steps	Write out schedule, who is speaking, topic to discuss
Asking for a promotion	Write a vision statement for yourself in the current job; synthesize the major hurdles you have overcome; abstract three principles as your value-add	List all job duties, describe how you completed each, outline your next major projects assigned

Integrated reasoning is the most cost effective method to advance your fluid intelligence at any age. There are no fees, no particular amount of time to set aside for practice. Integrated reasoning can be incorporated in your daily activities as a way of thinking to extract and express ideas.

Integrated reasoning will energize your thinking as well as increase the biological well-being of your brain. **Simply put, you are promoting your integrated reasoning intellect when you actively synthesize new meanings continually.** What this means is you construct new meanings from the vast data you are consuming, then you update ideas constantly by reconciling, interpreting, and converting these concepts, ideas, approaches, and solutions within the context of your vast existing experience and knowledge. Integrated reasoning is a dynamic cognitive brain habit where ideas are rarely static. You are exercising your integrated reasoning when you:

- form uncommon ideas.
- identify new problems.
- generate and revise workable solutions.
- reject or accept possible directions.

Integrated reasoning requires that you pool information from a handful of reliable sources, combine the key ideas, and condense the core meanings to their bare essence. Note that I say "handful," because often too many sources are perused, but only at a shallow level. For frontal lobe strengthening, It's better to go deeper when processing a few meaningful sources than shallowly processing many sources.

In relaying transformed information to others, do not start with the minutiae—from the bottom up. You will lose their attention if you have them go through the same arduous process of sifting through the large volumes of data. Start with the big ideas instead; it is more mind captivating for you and for those with whom you are communicating.

Being a CEO (Chief Entrepreneur Officer), you want to lead by example. Show others how big ideas, new solutions, and new opportunities are created, generated, and pervasively incorporated at multiple levels of communication. How many times have you left a meeting and thought it was the biggest waste of time? Or hung up from a conference call and been exhausted by fast-fire exchange of undirected, low-level ideas with lack of meaningful takeaways or best next steps? Or gone to a lecture or community service meeting with high expectations but leaving in frustration due to the lack of a clear message?

> Transformative thinking does not start from nothing. For novelty to emerge, new ideas are rooted in old ones.

Reflect on your entrepreneur of ideas status:

- Look at your sent email (or text messages) and locate ten that you wanted to send and receive back meaningful messages. What percentage are formulaic and predictable in the messaging and what percentage show high-level integrated reasoned messages? Is the message noticeably written by you, or could it have been written by anyone? Does it bring together ideas that were previously discussed with new concepts? Is it perfunctory or inspiring? Now rewrite one message you wish you had sent. From this point forward, take the time to write abstract, meaningful messages when it matters. This is one easy way to regularly practice constructing big ideas.

- Think back about a gathering of friends you recently attended and whether or not you had a meaningful conversation with a single person there or if it was all scripted at a superficial level of engagement. Now, for an upcoming outing, make a concerted effort to discuss some topic in detail, particularly if you and the other party may have differing views.
- Do you daily share something you read or heard on the news and give specific ways that you would improve the situation? I hear all the time how much people disagree with this point of view or that point of view. But individuals rarely voice the rationale for their stand because they have not taken the time to get to a deeper level of understanding.

Integrated Reasoning: A Comparison

Contrast the two stories of Mark and Wesley below to gain a better handle on why integrated reasoning is the significant groundwork necessary for increasing brain edge.

Case 1: Mark, a competitive individual with ample integrated reasoning capacity

Mark started a new career at age sixty-three, an age when many of his friends were either retired or certainly thinking of retiring. His bold move into a new job summoned different knowledge and responsibilities from the skill sets of his previous jobs, requiring major readjustment and on-the-job training. A year into his new job, he decided to get a cognitive checkup, a BrainHealth Physical, not because he was worried, but because he was curious about what a benchmark of his core cognitive areas (i.e., strategic attention, integrated reasoning, and innovation) would tell him about his brain's function. Plus, he prided himself in proactively being in the know and was always seeking ways to challenge and improve his high-performance edge.

The outcome of his assessment revealed that he excelled on measures of integrated reasoning.

- Mark synthesized complex information into novel ideas. He absorbed and processed new, unfamiliar content and constructed original ideas that were not explicitly stated.
- Mark showed a rich capacity to efficiently encapsulate multiple rich interpretations and applications from complex information.
- Mark actively constructed new thoughts and meanings by linking ideas from his rich experience and knowledge to the new skills.
- Mark was not stuck in the concrete data, words, and ideas as explicitly presented, nor was he blocked or overwhelmed by the abundant unfamiliar data he was being asked to absorb.

Mark's high level capacity of integrated reasoning likely accounts for why he quickly rose to a pivotal national leadership position and was able to take on great challenges in his new career. Within a year after the job shift, he was energized and contributing new ideas and ways of thinking to his colleagues. He was able to dynamically employ strategies to blend his rich knowledge and experience base with new on-the-job responsibilities. He put into practice the habit of utilizing frontal lobe processes to continually synthesize vast information into new, broader ways of approaching critical decisions and tasks. Mark actively added to his intellectual savings account.

His brainpower was a **major** contribution to his Fortune 500 company and supports a potentially positive side of **brainomics,** the economic benefits from brain gain. Mark's brain was being strengthened and the corporation's bottom line was likely boosted.

Case 2: Wesley, a competitive individual but with fledgling integrated reasoning capacity

When I saw Wesley, he was a fifty-two-year-old executive who had been a stockbroker. Wesley's performance on integrated reasoning tasks during his BrainHealth Physical was well below average. His primary way to absorb content entailed condensing and rearranging the content, paraphrasing the same ideas into his own words, and repeating the key points. He did not transform information into novel or generalized ideas other than those already conveyed. Although Wesley was skillfully competent at reducing the vast information he was given, he did little to change and construct broader perspectives.

Wesley had lost his job due to restructuring and was struggling to find a path to translate his old skills to a new job. Even though he was extremely bright, hardworking, and competitive, he was unable to create ways to reframe his vast expertise and knowledge to fit a changing, demanding environment.

On the surface, one might quickly conclude that Mark is smarter than Wesley. I would argue that this is not the case; in fact, they are both well above average intelligence. Mark, however, has used his brain dynamically to make it work smarter, which has paid off and will continue to pay off in the long run. Wesley, on the other hand, needs to ramp up his integrated reasoning capacity; it takes concerted effort, increasing challenges, and regular practice. Mark has continued to build this pivotal brain function at each decade. Wesley has not fully activated and harnessed his brainpower.

> Become a masterful synthesizer; don't remain an apprentice.

Our brain is designed to be a great synthesizer, but it requires effort to keep this amazing feat fine-tuned. Our brain is expertly capable of boiling down massive input streaming in and transforming ideas into generalized, abstracted essences of new meanings, new directions, new patterns of operating. The worrisome trend is that despite our brain being preferentially biased to extract meaning from the continuous, immense input; its synthesizing adeptness is rapidly losing ground.

> Ramping up your integrated reasoning will increase your brainpower. Exploit your capacity to design new knowledge, unveil new discoveries, chart new paths, and even invent new ways of thinking about old issues.

The problem is individuals are spending less and less time building, strengthening, and maintaining this platinum brain asset of integrated reasoning. Ramping up your integrated reasoning will increase your brainpower. We are weakening our brain's capacity to be a great synthesizer by overwhelming it with too much data and distracting information. We are constantly besieging our brain with information through all sensory inputs—visual, auditory, olfactory, tactile, and kinesthetic. As we take in, manage, and appraise vast amounts of information from every information platform possible—from conversations to computers to phones to television to newspapers, magazines, and books—we are incessantly processing thousands of stimuli and ideas, little to which we should pay conscious attention.

> Without practice, integrated reasoning capacity does not thrive or even survive regardless of how smart you are.

Catapult your Brain Plasticity: Utilize Your Complex Mental Capacity

Breakthrough brain discoveries reveal strong evidence as to what:

- Drives brain fitness
- Derails brain fitness

The answers lie largely in utilization issues. A common theme throughout this book is that **you control the destiny of your brain health.** Now consider this: how you use or fail to use your frontal lobe's complex thinking capacity of integrated reasoning drives whether you achieve and maintain higher levels of brain fitness or, conversely, whether you lose and regress to lower levels, at any age.

The following findings will hopefully give you the fuel you need to commit to a brain health exercise program this very day so you don't lose one more day of your brain's potential. In a randomized study of the effects of complex mental activity on brain and cognitive plasticity, my team and I found that engaging in integrated reasoning for a relatively short period of time was associated with **significant brain changes:**[1]

- Increases in brain blood flow by as much as 12 percent. This news alone should arouse you to invest in your brain by adopting complex thinking workouts daily. A healthy brain's total blood flow **decreases** each decade beginning at age twenty. The evidence of increasing brain blood flow with complex mental activity indicates that not only can you increase the total blood flow to build a healthier brain, but you can also prevent the inevitable reduction. When you engage in complex thinking, your brain's neurons demand glucose and oxygen, which therefore increases blood flow. Bottom line: the earlier you start and the longer you continue to engage in complex mental activity, the more you are likely improving your brain's health.

- Strengthening of communication between vital brain regions—specifically the left hippocampal region in the temporal lobe, which is linked to memory and learning, and the left inferior frontal lobe, which is linked to higher-order reasoning and problem solving.
- Structural brain changes that connect the parahippocampus region to the frontal lobe region of the brain.
- Marked improvements in frontal lobe cognitive functions, both those trained as well as many that were not specifically trained.

> Your brain may be sleepwalking through your days when you use your mind as a massive storage bin. Take the brain challenge to continually engage in complex mental activities.

The results are powerful. After six to twelve weeks of engaging in complex integrating reasoning, research participants demonstrated (1) cognitive gains, (2) increased brain blood flow, (3) improvements in brain efficiency, and (4) structural changes in white matter connections. This scientific evidence clearly shows that you can and do neuroengineer your brain by how you use it. Do not take this responsibility lightly. Make increasing your frontal lobe power your mission right now.

Brainomics Movement and You

My goal is to motivate you to join a brainomics movement to engage in complex mental activity. Why? Complex mental activity:

- reduces cognitive declines and losses.
- reverses degenerative brain changes.
- builds cognitive reserves.
- makes neurons healthier, at a molecular and cellular level.
- creates a smarter, longer-lasting brain.

The impact of weakened integrated reasoning capacity will dramatically increase the cost burden as generations age, thus negatively impacting brainomics. Weakened integrated reasoning is slowly robbing our intellectual capital, personally and societally.

> You cannot afford to let your integrated reasoning capacity atrophy.

How to Enhance Integrated Reasoning

Refocus your brain and sharpen your integrated reasoning capacity. The sooner you start, the better for long-term brain health. You can take advantage of the brain's smart design to create new ideas and tackle tough, never before experienced problems. Knowing practice makes perfect, expend major efforts toward building your brain's software to flexibly move from the known to the unknown, extracting the core messages. A high-performance brain can quickly combine seemingly disparate pieces of information to produce generalized principles while knowing expeditiously what to ignore.

Brain science and your prefrontal cortex guides you in reviewing the issues of each day, as well as problem finding—not just problem solving. Integrated reasoning calls upon the prefrontal cortex to combine existing experience with new happenings to search out and identify problems before they happen. Much of what your brainpower allows you to achieve is futurist thinking—not just reactionary thinking.

> Regardless of age, you can be a synthesizer and generator of new ideas and issues to be solved—energizing your brain.

Think about talking with your boss, brainstorming at a board meeting, seeking medical advice from your doctor, or probing for wiser investment practices from a financial advisor. What if you only absorbed the ideas you heard exactly as they were presented, without reprocessing to discern how it fits with your personal knowledge, biases, and experiences? You would be like a senseless brain guppy, taking in information without adding any insight or putting the new input into the perspective of your unique point of view. Not surprisingly, the chances of retaining information in this un-combined, rote way are very low—not to mention it is a wasted brain investment.

A better brain habit to adopt is to practice synthesizing ideas into one or two abstracted statements when presented with information. Ask probing questions that push the envelope on deeper thinking and action. For example, before going in to a meeting with your colleagues, boss, or volunteer organization, ask yourself: What changes do I want or what crucial issue do I need their help solving? What do I want them to consider? What are desired outcomes from this discussion? After a meeting, write down consolidated ideas, asking yourself: What are some new take-home messages? How does my thinking before the meeting compare with my thinking afterward? How can I use new information to redirect and reset goals? Write a synthesized brief of the meeting in three to five sentences and send it to those you met with to let them know you were listening and that the ideas and time they contributed made a difference. In doing so, you take pause and strategically engage your frontal lobe to reason continuously. Pushing your brainpower of integrated reasoning will be a boon to your brain health and your brain efficiency. It will help you think smarter, not harder.

Boost your brainpower: Stretch and challenge your mind to construct deeper-level, thought-filled ideas when presented with any type of information (magazine articles, movies, books, television shows, lectures, sermons, songs, political speeches, physician reports, comic strips, jokes, emails, etc.).

Extensive brain practices will help you:

1. ask probing questions about the unknown.
2. offer new possibilities to advance ideas and projects.
3. determine new paths that fit with your life changes.

A client exercised his integrated reasoning skills when he told me this new insight he gleaned after a talk I gave: "Your message of the importance of a deeper level of thinking—to find the pearl in what one is hearing, reading, seeing, etc.—was *profound*. I have always wanted to learn the details so I could be accurate. Now I realize that has kept my thinking at a fairly superficial level. Not good for a healthy, stimulated frontal lobe! Thanks for the eye and mind opener."

Integrated Reasoning Exercises

Integrated reasoning is a brain habit that should become your blueprint to absorb and repurpose content. The more often you practice this habit, the more intellectual capital you will build.

The best ways to practice integrated reasoning are to:

- take in the new meanings and quickly move away from the literal meanings conveyed.
- adroitly combine the diverse ideas with previous experiences.
- generate novel interpretations that few would have conceived.
- combine concepts—new with old—to help you harness your highest level of integrated reasoning capacity.

Try improving your fluid intelligence and increasing your intellectual capital in the integrated reasoning practice tasks below.

Practice Task #1:
Read this T. Boone Pickens quote: *"If you're going to run with the big dogs, you have to get out from under the porch."*

1. Give three explanations for what this saying could mean.
2. Relate one or two events in your life to this principle.

When you begin to think of how to encapsulate and convey your thoughts into higher-level concepts, your messages will be more meaningful. Being able to translate complex ideas into simple examples represents one of the highest levels of intellectual thinking.

Practice Task #2:
Think back on one of your favorite movies or books from the past year.

1. Generate five to eight different take-home messages that could be gleaned from the movie or book.
2. Moving forward, which lesson would influence your life the most and why?

Instead of simply retelling the plotline of a movie or book, practice your integrated reasoning skills. Brainstorm with others who also saw the movie or read the book and share your ideas. This builds deeper-level thinking. We have libraries full of books in our homes and oftentimes cannot remember whether we have read a book or not because we read it superficially. **Reading as an isolated activity without deeper processing will not build brainpower.**

The above activities challenge your mind and boost your brainpower. Practicing constructing high-level, generalized, and abstracted meaning allows you to move beyond the details to the bigger picture. Pushing your mind to constantly synthesize meanings is a lot of work, but the cost in effort pays off increasing your brain's robustness and the power of your frontal lobe functions. The more you make such mind stretching a habit, the easier it will become over time.

Integrated reasoning helps you identify key messages to inspire different groups or audiences, reduce complex material down to its memorable essence, relate current and future broad impact issues, and tune in to insightful generalizations to chart new directions.

To build brainpower requires integrated reasoning to increase intellectual capital.

There are three strategies that will help you enhance your integrated reasoning, thus improving your frontal lobe function and brain efficiency. They are:

- Zoom In
- Zoom Out
- Zoom Deep and Wide

The Brainpower of Zoom In

It is a false belief to think that you are either a big-picture thinker or a detail-oriented person. You cannot be a big-picture thinker without knowing the supporting facts or else you would be an empty suit. **The brainpower of zoom in** requires attending to facts, content, and the situation at hand. Gathering facts and using them to support a novel approach is essential to enhancing integrated reasoning and deeper level thinking. However, it's a delicate balance of knowing when to gather more information and knowing when to stop looking for more facts to develop a point of view. **The key is to toggle back and forth from the immense raw details to form high-level ideas.** It is not enough to understand all the facts; it is highly critical to fit them into a larger schema.

> The whole is more than the sum of its parts.

The Brainpower of Zoom Out

We often cannot see the forest for the trees. We listen to political or graduation speeches and may remember funny one-liners or embarrassing moments shared, but we often fail to appreciate any meaningful or generalized messages that are typically conveyed. To be able to glean synthesized messages requires the **brainpower of zoom out,** to see a broader perspective, to appreciate the big picture. It is important to harness the **brainpower of zoom out** and lift off to a helicopter view, assessing pieces of data and disparate viewpoints from above, merging them into the major themes, core concepts, and broad principles. Consolidating facts and opinions into big ideas and perspectives is necessary to cultivate creative thinking and problem solving. **The brainpower of zoom out helps avoid silos of isolated or static thinking.**

The Brainpower of Zoom Deep and Wide

The **brainpower of zoom deep and wide** is the cognitive strategy of incorporating the major principles and generalized lessons learned into broader applications. This is cognitive strategy transfer at its best. **The brainpower of zoom deep and wide requires the deepest level of thinking where you apply novel developments from one area to other issues, other problems.**

Zoom deep and wide represents:

- Synthesized topics to guide effective meetings and gatherings
- Generalized applications to mentor new trainees, colleagues, and family members
- Intellectually energized writing in emails, speeches, and projects

The dynamic ability to assimilate information from multiple sources to apply to diverse, novel, and complex issues requires the integrated reasoning strategy of zoom deep and wide. It is critical to solving new problems that have ambiguity or arise unexpectedly almost daily. If you immediately knew the answer to a problem, then that situation would not be defined as a problem. Fine-tuning integrated reasoning capacity through practice equips individuals with the cognitive tools to discover and develop improved solutions to emerging problems, including analyzing information that may not even be available to them based on prior learning.

Practice Task #3:

Exercise your integrated reasoning talents by synthesizing the following quote from Steve Jobs. Use the brainpower of zoom deep and wide.

A lot of people in our industry haven't had very diverse experiences. So they don't have enough dots to connect, and they end up with very linear solutions without a broad perspective on the problem. The broader one's understanding of the human experience, the better design we will have.

The cognitive finesse involved in increasing aptitude in **zooming deep and wide** is exceptionally complex and requires heavy brain lifting. Most people easily give up and only identify the generalized ideas from specific readings or meetings—failing to creatively adapt these new concepts to inform new ways of thinking and acting. High performers know their area of expertise, build on it, and efficiently engage this knowledge to advance innovation across domains. Think of it as a mathematic equation.

$$A + B = Ø$$

A=incoming content, B=knowledge/experience,
Ø = meaning converted into a new, transformed approach or product

Practice Task #4:

Planning for an upcoming important meeting based on previous gatherings requires dynamic toggling across all three brainpowers of zooming—**zoom in** to the issues at hand; **zoom out** to the broadest perspectives to see vast solutions and potential directions, and **zoom deep and wide** to figure out new framing for old problems and novel applications to proven practices.

1. Write and distribute ahead of time the target topics to discuss or problem solve from the previous meetings.
2. Before the meeting takes place, think through what success would look like when the meeting is over.
3. Identify what topics attendees should think about or papers to read before the meeting. Have the meeting members consider the abstract ideas—not just give silos of opinions. The more prepared they are, the more they will be brain engaged in the discussion.
4. Lead from the bottom up. Let attendees take active thought-roles, as it will help to challenge and hone their frontal lobe skills as opposed to when the leader is always in charge of the meeting.

5. Identify and challenge new perspectives (zoom out) and rationale (zoom in) for high level goals, not information downloading.

6. Develop novel approaches to solve the primary key problems and apply proven practices to new contexts.

Meetings are one of the greatest brain drains in the workplace. Think of the number of people attending, their salaries, and the cost when nothing or next to nothing is accomplished. Practicing the skill of integrated reasoning will help create meetings that stretch the minds and build the brains of those attending and increase individual and corporate intellectual capital.

Practice Task #5:
Read the "Great Balls of Fire" text below to complete this next exercise. I want you to see how different it feels if you read it with two different goals in mind. First, I want you to read it with the idea that you will be tested on how many of the facts you can recite back after reading it.

Reading for the details will keep you in a mind-set focused on the pieces of information without thinking of how the pieces of information might be connected to more than that conveyed by the text.

Second, read "Great Balls of Fire" with the goal of formulating which of its lessons are still relevant today. The more knowledge one has, the easier the second reading becomes. Whatever the age, when you engage the brain to be open to constructing new meanings, you will always be more turned on to learning than when requiring the brain to be a robotic absorber and recorder of mass content.

"Great Balls of Fire" by Abul-Fazl*
(Accessed from *Lapham's Quarterly*)

Superficial observers look upon polo as a mere amusement and consider it only play, but men of more exalted views see in it a means of learning promptitude and decision. It tests the value of a man and strengthens the bonds of friendship. Strong men learn in playing this game the art of riding, and the animals learn to perform feats of agility and to obey the reins. Hence His Majesty Akbar the Great is very fond of this game. Externally, the game adds to the splendor of his court, but viewed from a higher point, it reveals concealed talents.

When His Majesty goes to the field in order to play this game, he selects an opponent and some active and clever players, who are only filled with one thought, namely, to show their skill against the opponents of His Majesty. From motives of kindness, His Majesty never orders anyone to be a player, but chooses the pairs by the cast of the die. There are not more than ten players, but many more keep themselves in readiness. When twenty-four minutes have passed, two players take rest, and two others supply their place.

His Majesty is unrivaled for the skill which he shows in the various ways of hitting the ball; he often manages to strike the ball while in the air and astonishes all. When a ball is driven to a goal, they beat the kettledrum, so that all who are far and near may hear it. In order to increase the excitement, betting is allowed. The players win from each other, and he who brought the ball to the goal wins most.

His Majesty also plays polo on dark nights, which caused much astonishment, even among clever players. The balls which are used at night are set on fire. For this purpose palás wood is used, which is very light and burns for a long time. For the sake of adding splendor to the games, which is necessary in wordly matters, His Majesty has knobs of gold and silver fixed to the tops of the polo sticks. If one of them breaks, any player that gets hold of the pieces may keep them.

*Abul-Fazl, from The Institutes of Akbar. Abul-Fazl served as a historian and secretary to Emperor Akbar, reforming Islamic theological practices and becoming a military commander of southern India in 1599. Following a rebellion by Akbar's son, Abul-Fazl was ordered back to court but was intercepted and assassinated en route. In addition to his historical works, the author is said to have translated the Bible into Persian.

Now that you have read the "Great Balls of Fire" two times, answer these queries:

1. What are ten major themes you deciphered from "Great Balls of Fire"?
2. How many generalized messages can you generate?

3. Apply those meanings to three different current world situations.

Some of you may be thinking, "This seems like being in school again. I do not want to think that hard." But what is vital to keep in mind is that if you desire to stretch your brain years to more closely align and match your life span, then these brain habits can and will make a difference.

Some themes from "Great Balls of Fire" might be:

- Compassion
- Fairness
- Encouragement
- Motivation
- Competition
- Excellence
- Inclusion
- Passion

Some generalized messages might be:

- Team building around freedom.
- Games are a way to bring joy to dark times.
- Recognize physical and mental limits.
- Competition amplifies talent.
- One must lead by example.
- Preparation and chance provide an opportunity.

When you challenge your brain to synthesize individualized interpretations from incoming information, you will be building stronger frontal lobe networks—networks important for staying brain fit longer and building brain reserves at every age.

> You can rewire your frontal lobe connectivity by constantly thinking in challenging, complex ways.

The goal is to optimize the core mental processes of strategic attention (as discussed in the previous chapter), integrated reasoning, and innovation (see the next chapter) for a sustainable brain future that supports your ability to make vital decisions every day. The more frequently you push your brain to absorb meaning by using the brainpower of zooming in, out, and deep and wide, the more efficiently your brain will work.

Boost your brainpower: Make a concerted effort to transform your hundreds of thoughts each day to the highest level of thinking as possible.

The brainpower of zooming is not a trivial skill; it is recognized as a vital cognitive skill that has not been easy to assess. A recent survey of 740 business faculty worldwide revealed that they believed incoming business students needed to assimilate, interpret, and convert data, evaluate outcomes, and listen—key skills for twenty-first-century students and future leaders in business.[2] Armed with that data, the Graduate Management Admission Council (GMAC) reformatted and added a new section to the Graduate Management Admission Test (GMAT). The title of the new section: "Integrated Reasoning."

According to the announcement from GMAC, which leads the development of the GMAT, "The new integrated reasoning section of the GMAT will be a microcosm of today's b-school classroom." Dave Wilson, president and CEO of GMAC, went on to say, "These questions will provide critical intelligence to schools about the ability of prospective students to make sound decisions by evaluating, assimilating or extrapolating data."

Integrated Reasoning Linked to Strategic Leadership

Integrated reasoning is one of our most complex and forceful thinking capacities that can be enhanced. As such, this skill is associated with decisive and strategic leadership.

William Duggan shares his definitions of three kinds of intuition—ordinary, expert, and strategic—in his book *Strategic Intuition: The Creative Spark in Human Achievement*.[3] He defines each type of intuition:

- Ordinary intuition is a gut instinct.
- Expert intuition is a snap judgment that is done at rapid speed, based on experience.
- Strategic intuition is a slow, thoughtful way of solving a problem.

I can see the parallels between intuition and integrated reasoning. Precisely,

- Zoom out is a quickly abstracted idea. This is similar to a gut instinct, a vague notion of the key points and directions.
- Zoom in corresponds to the power of knowledge where one can make a very quick, snap judgment or decision based on extensive facts and expertise.
- Zoom deep and wide is a process that is not fast, but it is deliberate. It involves an effortful, integrative process of reflective thinking through all the possibilities. Strategic leaders will use this type of cognitive process to prime new ideas and advance lines of thinking, as well as rethink past misdirection. This is the foundation for entrepreneurial and innovative thinking that is discussed in the next chapter.

When honed, the benefits of integrated reasoning and strategic global thinking spill over to many frontal lobe and other brain functions. The ability to harness this global perspective is fundamental to creative thinking, problem solving, and energizing productivity.

Remember Linda, the high-level executive at a Fortune 500 company who was interested in maximizing her cognitive performance? For her, learning and applying the brainpowers of zooming to her everyday life, both personally and professionally, has led to increased productivity. "Zooming in, zooming out, and zooming deep and

Brain value of integrated reasoning
- Become a mastermind of information
- Create fresh and bigger ideas rather than crank out rote facts
- Chart unique insights by combining new data with rich experiences and knowledge

wide has advanced my brain potential. Zooming deep and wide is a skill I had not cultivated to any degree, but now I'm finding that using it leads to better work, particularly on the most challenging assignments like strategy development. The statements I prepare are more thought filled and forward thinking than the ones I prepared last year."

The brainpower of zooming encourages deliberate, reflective thinking, not just a snap judgment or acting on a gut reaction. Using this strategic approach to understanding information in your daily life requires dynamically shifting from what is in front of you to a global view and transcending the literal surface to construct novel and deeper levels of meaning in contexts you never before experienced. Integrated reasoning is a platinum cognitive asset that you absolutely can enhance to increase your performance and boost your intellectual capital.

Integrated reasoning allows you to identify and group important details into condensed, global meanings; thereby efficiently limiting the massive amounts of information one has to manipulate, comprehend, encode, and recall. My research has shown that when individuals improve their ability to assimilate and synthesize information, they experience a direct beneficial effect on brain health fitness.[4-5] There is an added bonus to keeping the frontal lobe skill of integrated reasoning in shape: if exercised and maintained into late life, integrated reasoning significantly improves and spills over to other executive cognitive functions that were never trained, achieving gains in higher memory for details and faster speed of processing.

> Practice the brainpower of zooming to strengthen integrated reasoning continually to make your brain think smarter—longer.

Benefits of integrated reasoning intensive workouts	
↑ Mental productivity	↓ Brain fatigue
↑ Brain energy	↓ Brain boredom
↑ Idea innovation	↓ Rote repetition

Move out of a rote-mill way of idea processing to churning out newly created ideas. Integrated reasoning alone does not maximize your cognitive prowess, but it is fundamental to creative thinking, problem solving, and energized productivity. Learn more about the brainpower of innovation and mental flexibility in the next chapter to build even more cognitive capacity.

Know Brainers

1. Harness the dynamic brainpowers of zooming
   - Zoom In:
     Get the facts.
   - Zoom Out:
     Transform literal facts into bigger ideas, diverse perspectives, and global themes by combining new input with existing knowledge.
   - Zoom Deep and Wide:
     Formulate broader novel applications with bold, deep, more strategic thinking.
2. Rewire your brain's frontal lobe connectivity by deeper level thinking.
3. Transform your habitual thinking and acting by constantly synthesizing and constructing abstracted meanings that are useful—not random.
4. Recognize when you are engaging in rote versus riveting communication of ideas or planning something that is original.
5. Mentor your team members to become CEOs (aka Cognitive Entrepreneur Officers) of their own thinking, contributing new ways to change current practices on their own by exploring new concepts, modifying, transforming, extending, and even rejecting current thinking patterns.
6. Knowledge is power when it is not static but when it is constantly being updated by combining new possibilities with rich experiences.

For additional tools and tips visit makeyourbrainsmarter.com.

CHAPTER 6

INNOVATE TO INSPIRE YOUR THINKING

Do you want to be smarter and more creative?
What limits your innovative thinking capacity?
What tasks inspire creativity and which ones just need to be completed?
What is the fuel to engage your brain's strongest creative power?
Can you train your brain to be innovative and imaginative?

As a society, we believe that we are able to innovate best during youth, a fertilized and frenetic life stage when creativity is encouraged. However, as we age, imaginative thinking is all too often ignored, fatigued, and underdeveloped. It is incorrect to think that not much can be done to increase your creative prowess. So when does innovation and creativity peak?

Our complex frontal lobe networks are the creative epicenters of our brains as well as the command centers of our lives. Everyone has the potential to break new ground, to be more inventive at any age. One obstacle to our doing so is receiving an early label that inaccurately frames our brain and robs us of our confidence. A second is the widely held belief that limits the age expectations of when we can be creative geniuses.

Definition: Innovation is the ability to generate and exploit new ideas to solve problems; to seek, devise, and employ improved ways of dealing with unknown and unfamiliar contexts; or to create something that is original and valuable.

- Innovation is about improving upon and changing old ways of doing things through novel thinking.
- Innovative thinkers practice mental flexibility—stretching their creativity and imagination.
- Ingenious thinkers are open to experimentation to rethink practices and are at ease with ambiguity.
- Innovators are not beaten down by failure, rather, they constantly ask what they can learn from their mistakes.

"Imagination is more important than knowledge. Knowledge is limited. Imagination encircles the world." —Einstein

An Innovator

Clint Bruce is an innovator. He owns his own company, started a successful non-profit, and is a former Navy SEAL. In any meeting, conversation, or communication with him, your mind will be stretched—as he challenges you to think about new ideas and new ways to approach situations that were not even on your radar or in your repertoire of thoughts. Was he born this way? Or was his innovative mind built because of his experience as a Navy SEAL whose team's survival depended on his ability to quickly see reality and make the impossible happen?

When I first met Clint, he complained that his brain was firing so rapidly that he could not slow it down. After brain health training, Clint is armed with the strategies he needs to implement in order to constantly solve new problems, to explore new possibilities. Clint's innovative training regimen is simple. My team challenged Clint to strengthen his already stellar innovative capacity. With every task put before him, whether with his family, at the office, or when consulting across the country, Clint seeks, devises, and employs improved ways of dealing with unknown and unfamiliar contexts. He thrives on tough problems to solve. When you have a conversation with him, you can see his prodigious brainpower of innovation in action.

Are you an innovator?

You can ramp up your innovative capacity.

The destiny of your innovative thinking capacity is largely in your hands. Your innovative capacity is limitless, and your only enemy is yourself. We often think our most imaginative years are behind us. Some believe you either have it or you don't. Others think creativity has to be nourished by a certain age or else it's too late. And others still think it's in your genetic code.

You can spark creativity in your brain and stoke the smoldering fire of your imaginative capacity at any age. Innovation can be fostered and developed no matter your life's work; creativity can be trained and regained if you practice and unlock its immense capacity to create and innovate.

Creative versus Smart

Research reveals that people who are smart or have high general intelligence are not necessarily the same as those who are highly creative.[1-2] Of course, the question of whether you would wish to be smarter or more creative is a bit of an esoteric academic exercise. But we often place a demarcation between being smart and being creative as if they are separate entities. This separation insinuates that if you are smart, you may or may not be creative and vice versa.

Webster's Thesaurus has very different synonyms to describe the two. Synonyms for "creative" include:

clever . . . inspired . . . inventive . . . ingenious . . . prolific . . . visionary . . . stimulating.

Synonyms for "smart" consist of words like:

adept . . . . apt . . . brilliant . . . knowing . . . sharp . . . shrewd . . . wise

The difference in meanings conveys a sense that being smart is a *state,* and being creative is an *action.* For me, these words can be used synonymously, and I will use these words interchangeably throughout this book. All too often we think of "creative" in the context of the arts and innovation in science—which is a major mistake. **Innovation and creativity matter at every life stage, for every walk of life.** You can experience an increase in brainpower when you constantly practice being an entrepreneur of ideas.

I have polled people to find out their beliefs on how they value creativity by asking: "Would you rather be smarter or more creative?" Think about the question for yourself. What would you rather be? I've asked many individuals of different ages, genders, and backgrounds. The responses are fascinating.

One young executive said, "Well if they are mutually exclusive, then
I would rather be smart to allow myself to make better life and
business decisions. The term 'starving artist' must be at least
partially based in reality."
A thirtysomething female said, "Being creative leads to being smart
since creativity leads to new thoughts, truths, and ideas."
When I asked my twentysomething son, he said, "You need a level of
smart to be creative. There has to be a balance in levels of creativity
and smartness. If you are very creative and not very smart, you
might not have direction."
A female from the boomer generation responded saying, "Knowledge or
smarts is good, but being able to apply or talk about what I know
in a creative way is what can inspire, motivate, and educate. I
want to be more creative!"
A fortysomething male responded by saying, "I'd rather be more creative.
I already have a high IQ, but I'm too concrete at times. I'd rather
think out of the box more easily."

In actuality, both creative capacity and smartness work hand in hand to energize the brain. The ability to continually engage in innovative thinking is likely a key indicator of who will retain their smart capacity, the ability to acquire and build new knowledge.

Knowledge is part of the creative equation; we cannot go to the next level without knowing the basic facts. However, innovative thinking should work synergistically with analytical and practical thinking for the best results. Often we take in information as truth rather than pondering what we do not know. Nor do we consider how we can add or modify that knowledge or practice.

> *"Creativity is not just a matter of thinking in a certain way, but rather it is an attitude toward life."*
> —Robert Sternberg, a leading American psychologist and researcher

Your Innovative Capacity

However, innovation as a skill becomes paralyzed from lack of use, limited challenges, and fear of failure. Do not let your innovative capacity go dormant and weak from not being properly exercised. Below are innovation's greatest enemies:

- A brain on automatic pilot
- An avoidance of new challenges
- A belief that your best and most creative work is behind you
- An opposition to being renewable, adaptable
- A strong separation from those who have radically different viewpoints
- An evasion of collaborations on major projects

Innovation, creativity, and imagination require practice, just like staying proficient in a foreign language you once learned to speak. You are well aware that the less you use the second language, the weaker it gets. With total neglect over a span of years, you have to almost start from scratch to build the expertise to speak a foreign language fluently. The same is true for being innovative.

> Your brainpower of innovative thinking should be exercised daily.

If you have not been stretching your innovative skills, then now is the time to jump-start this immense brain capacity. How often do you:

- figure out ways to deal with new circumstances?
- adapt quickly and adeptly to novel challenges?
- shake up regular meetings that tend to drain the brain?
- break with past habits?

Reflect on your own capacity to be innovative in everyday tasks or ask someone who knows you well. I recently asked my son if he thought I was relatively smarter or more creative. He was too naive to realize this was a loaded question and answered instantly, "You are higher on the smart than creative scale, without question."

After I licked my wounds, he said, "I guess you didn't like my answer." I responded by explaining that I had to be innovative to do what I do and by always modifying and updating the research initiatives I encountered—always going in new directions. This immediately changed his mind, and he went on to say that he thought I had grown more creative over the past decade as I created and retooled the vision and expansion of brain discoveries at the Center for BrainHealth. I think he is correct; as a young adult, I was more interested in acquiring knowledge. Now I am energized by creating knowledge.

> Innovation drives national economic growth and well-being.

Innovative Thinkers Invent Again and Again

Dr. Alan Leshner, CEO of the American Association for the Advancement of Science and executive publisher of *Science* magazine, wrote an editorial titled, "Innovation Needs Novel Thinking."[3] He challenged funders to foster innovative research by encouraging scientists through the support of creative pursuits, instead of the already-know-the-answer line of research that is commonly practiced. I would elaborate on this to say **we need to train people—at every stage of life—to ignite their highest level of novel thinking.** This brain competency predominates as a key investment to enhance your intellectual capital.

You may be thinking to yourself: "Gee, I'm too old to start ramping up my innovative capacity now," or "Why should I start now when I just retired?" The greatest hindrance to enhancing your capacity of innovative thinking is your own self-limiting brain habits. We often desire that all days and projects be clearly delineated, in an almost cut-and-paste routine with as little deviation as possible. We get distressed rather than inspired when asked to rethink a project or action or mistake. My goal is to inspire you to break these brain-draining habits.

Many conceive brain aging as a relentless decline. Brain imaging studies support this view with evidence of age-related declines in the medial prefrontal cortex and deep brain structures. Corresponding with these brain losses are documented cognitive declines in innovative thinking and mental flexibility.[4] Does this sound like an impossible course to correct?

> The downward spiral of innovative brain decline can be changed, but it requires your commitment.

Frontal Lobe Connectivity Supports Innovative Thinkers

A neuroscientific team from Japan was among the first to document that individuals with higher innovative thinking scores also show increased structural connectivity between the frontal lobe and the corpus callosum—a deep portion of the brain that links both hemispheres. This research supports my view that the frontal lobe is positively related to pivotal dimensions of creativity—specifically cognitive flexibility.

Studies of brain efficiency are shedding light on the concept that more brain activation versus less is associated with more learning as a novice. When your brain becomes an expert, it works more efficiently. That is, those with higher expertise, perhaps associated with greater practice, perform the task more efficiently, with less brain activation.

> A more efficient brain does not have to work as hard.

Brain plasticity studies offer high promise that the declining brain capacity can be positively altered in the healthy brain by exercising innovative thinking. Findings show that the process of learning or creating something new is linked to changes in brain structure.[5] Stop and think for a moment: learning or creating something new is linked to changes in brain structure!

Your brain can be changed by how you use it, by how you activate it every day—no matter your age. Be astonished at what a powerful role you play in changing your brain.

Open up your thinking to devise new ways of doing things.

All of the core brainpowers—strategic attention, integrated reasoning, and innovation—require hard work. We falsely think we are either gifted in an area or not. But you can become more innovative if you take the challenge to heart and open your mind. You can become more creative and inventive with practice. You just need to recognize and fully embrace that you have the capacity to increase your genius.

The success of keeping your brainpower fully engaged throughout your life span depends largely on attending to and strengthening our immense innovative capacity. Each of us can strive to build an innovative brain, one that seeks ways to uncover the maximum number of possibilities. You need to use and therefore design your brain to move from the known to the unknown—but with foresight about the risks and opportunities that are changing at the speed of light.

Transformative Thinking

In my work with executive and high level management, I have found significant gains in innovative thinking after only six hours of concentrated brain training. Ninety-two percent of those trained showed improvements in generating new ideas. Before the training, their flexibility in deriving new ideas was restricted, concrete, and automatic. You might be thinking, "Of course they improved, you trained them!" However, the training was not dedicated to practicing this critical skill. The training provided the high level executives with the strategies needed

Become an entrepreneur of ideas.

to innovate. The bottom line: every individual has greater creative potential than they are currently achieving.

Nowhere has the significance of innovative thinking been more apparent than in the study of the brain. If cognitive neuroscience had not continued to challenge and seek alternative explanations for why some people show tremendous brainpower until late life while others seem halted in their early adulthood, we would still believe that decline is the only path our brains can take as we age. If scientists had not pushed to discover more about our most astonishing organ, we would not know that the brain can grow, change, and repair connections throughout life.

> Innovative brain building: Brain networks strengthen in response to new challenges or wither with status quo thinking at all ages.

I acknowledge that we are still unclear on exactly how to apply the knowledge from vast brain discoveries to real-life settings. But we do know enough to adopt better habits that will help our brains as we age. Remember, you have 100 billion neurons and trillions of deep brain connections working for you, waiting to be called on to strengthen your brainpower.

Take Advantage of Neuroplasticity

Your road to increasing innovation is rarely a straight line. Innovation and creativity are brain potentials that can be nurtured or stunted throughout life; they are lifelong processes, not a single stage or a goal reached.

Innovation has little to do with:

- How many hours you work
- How much information you absorb
- How many classes you take
- How many major tasks you design and complete
- How quickly you learn

> When imagination stalls, you are like the walking dead with little energy day by day.

So, how do you know if you are innovative or not? It's a matter of adopting nimble brain habits to energize your inner genius.

Building creativity requires continually exercising habits throughout your day, not simply every so often. Incite innovation daily when you:

- Seek to broaden and revamp your perspectives, to view life differently, by reading different types of books, exposing yourself to different types of people, changing routine work presentations, etc.
- Dismantle old linkages of information to allow new thoughts to brew
- Ponder free-flowing ideas
- Consciously and dedicatedly convert ideas into deliberate change
- Recognize there is no road map to get you there
- Reflect and learn from mistakes—quickly

However, it's not that you need to innovate at every moment, in every instance. Rather, you need to choose critical issues or messy problems to apply these abilities toward.

**To revolutionize your brainpower,
seek to be a change maker—now.**

Work, passion, and a sense of purpose are the best nourishments for healthy brain function and innovation. As I have said before, our brain is remarkable. We exhaust it each day, yet every morning we awake with a recharged battery, ready for the next challenge. And even though you can build your brain depending on how you use it every day, you must neuro-engineer it in the most engaging ways to stay inspired.

Remember Linda—the fiftysomething high-level executive of a Fortune 500 company? Linda was inherently very talented and an innovative thinker. She quickly broke through the glass ceiling at a very young age. Her insightful and innovative ways of thinking were obvious to all who worked with her. However, after years of climbing the ladder, she thought that she'd hit a plateau. "I felt frozen," she told me. The roadblock in her case was not her own inability to exercise innovative thinking but rather the environment in which she found herself. Her work environment championed and rewarded knowledge and constant output. Linda's environment was literally suffocating her creative power.

> **Boost your brainpower:** Step back and take note of how your environment is stifling and constraining your imagination. Instead of complaining—imagine, create, and develop potential solutions.

Innovative ideas are created out of fragments of information. Good, creative, and novel ideas are a composition of knowledge, experience, and new exposures fused in different ways.

Expand your extraordinary capacity for innovation by exercising the:

- Brainpower of infinite
- Brainpower of paradox
- Brainpower of unknown

> A bored brain is a brain in decline.

Brainpower of Infinite

Innovative ideas are created out of pieces of seemingly random data, recombined in such a novel way that the whole that was comprised of the pieces does not even look the same. There are infinite possibilities of how information can be connected in new ways to innovate. There is not a single answer or only one way to do things. Challenge your innovative capacity by practicing the **brainpower of infinite** strategy.

Practice Tasks:

1. Create novel and innovative topics in your email subject line.
2. If you give a lot of presentations or lead meetings, change the message and make it fresh each time. A stale talk will bore you the speaker/leader, and the audience will feel the zestless message.
3. In this tough economy, think of at least ten new ways you can cut your monthly budget by 30 percent. All too often, we complain but do not break new ground by breaking old habits to create a new modus operandi.
4. Mentor and encourage small teams to be inventive problem solvers on crucial projects.
5. Think of family gatherings that fall flat with the same old discussions. Stretch family members to engage in new ways they never have before, e.g., meet in new venues, discuss fascinating people of substance, or talk about current ethical dilemmas.
6. Buying the perfect gift for someone requires creativity and innovation. Watch what their preferences are and connect the observations to what you think they would want.

Brainpower of Paradox

Innovation and mental flexibility require embracing and learning from mistakes and challenges—overcoming insurmountable odds. Paradoxically, the tenacity to not get stopped or stuck by failure is the fuel that leads to the greatest advances in these areas. The **brainpower of paradox** is enhanced when one reflects on a completed task and perceives the holes, and then dynamically and flexibly reworks and reinvents for a better product/output. The mental flexibility required to reflect on, revisit, and seek better solutions engages the frontal lobe, optimizing learning, which leads to transformative new insights and fresh ways of approaching outdated tasks—large and small.

Practice Tasks:

1. Reflect on a meeting that was essentially a time waster. Think about how to re-engage the issues to bring about mutually beneficial solutions. Attempt to garner more participation and idea sharing to make gatherings more meaningful to attendees.
2. Rethink a project, presentation, or event that you think went well. Brainstorm at least five ways it could have gone even better and how it could be improved if you had another opportunity tomorrow.
3. Remember back on a happening that seemed like the worst possible turn of events for you at the time and list at least five good things that eventually arose from that challenge.
4. Identify your favorite mistake weekly and see what you can now learn by looking back.

Brainpower of Unknown

The **brainpower of unknown** requires valuing curiosity and asking, "What if?" We are born with an unparalleled capacity to explore. As we age, we often set our brains on default mode until they become paralyzed in familiarity. This is a choice, not a necessity. **A highly innovative person is never satisfied with the status quo (the known) and is always looking for ways to move to the unknown, where things are constantly improving, changing, growing, and expanding.**

Practice Tasks:

1. Volunteer to direct something you have never taken the lead on before; you will feel stretched with new ways of thinking.
2. When a new opportunity approaches you, think of ways it will teach you something new if you spend the time to be innovative.
3. When you are feeling overwhelmed by a new position or

major responsibility where 75 percent of what you are doing is unknown, practice earlier brainpowers:

a. Brainpower of two (see chapter 4)—identify your two most important tasks to learn to make the greatest difference in your new position in the next month.

b. Brainpower of zooming (see integrated reasoning, chapter 5)—step back to appreciate how the important task you identified above fits into a bigger picture while continually breaking down important new learning tasks into doable steps.

As you expand your inventiveness, write how you have or will attempt to manifest each high-powered skill to increase your intellectual capital.

• Cause new things to happen:

_____

• Switch to novel modes of thinking:

_____

• Energize out-of-the-box thinking:

_____

• Construct ideas that relate to the future:

_____

• Imagine how things can be beyond the situation:

_____

• Seek ways to improve processes and products:

_____

• Become an agent of peace in a difficult conflict within your sphere of influence

_____

Remember: when you are hunting your elephants (see chapter 4) on your daily to-do list, note one thing each day that you want to revisit, rethink, and reinvent. It is best if the one thing you revisit is an elephant and not a rabbit. Your brain will be energized as you begin to practice and amplify your fuller innovative potential.

> As you age, your brain gets better at envisioning and making the impossible happen—if you keep your inventiveness well-tuned.

Innovative thinking is pivotal to the upside of **brainomics**—the economic gains possible from advancing innovative thinking. Are you motivated to start today to practice and strengthen your innovative thinking?

Know Brainers

1. Your brainpower of innovation can be enhanced every year of your life.
2. Your brain is inspired when you seek as many diverse new ways to do old things.
3. Challenge your brainpower and increase your intellect by devising a wide array of original solutions and interpretations regularly.
4. Innovative thinking is like speaking a foreign language—it must be practiced to stay strong and become more dependable.
5. Your brain's connectivity is enhanced when you engage in mentally innovative thinking.
6. If you never thought of yourself as an innovative thinker, it is never too late to start and improve by incremental degrees.
7. Even small incremental improvements in innovative thinking could contribute to your bottom line.
8. Your innovative capacity is limited primarily by you.
9. The more you push yourself to identify and apply diverse strategies to solve problems, the more likely you will transfer this skill to other areas of your brain function.

SECTION III

MAKE YOUR BRAIN SMARTER AT ANY AGE

The frontal lobe fitness needs of the millennial generation vary from those of the traditionalist generation. Baby boomers require still different frontal lobe practice as they begin navigating through their fifties and sixties. Building effective and efficient brain health levels across the life span requires an understanding of the basic needs of each one. Chapters 7 through 10 give specific case illustrations and tips based on cutting-edge neuroscience research for each generation.

CHAPTER 7

THE IMMEDIATES, 13–24 YEARS OF AGE

Y ou are an ImMEDIAte if you are currently between thirteen and twenty-four years of age. If you are an Immediate, your life blood is your *media*. I labeled this generation the ImMEDIAtes because you crave immediate access to your social network and are constantly satisfying your perpetual need to be connected.

Why is now the most vulnerable brain stage of your life?
What are the pros and cons of your amazing ability to stay hyperconnected?
Why is the Immediate generation slower to emerge into adulthood than earlier generations?
What is robbing you of your intellectual potential as an Immediate?
How can you conquer the obstacles that are slowing, perhaps even stalling, your frontal lobe fitness?
How do you catapult your brainpower to take advantage of your current stage of rapid frontal lobe development?
Can you unlock your creative potential when you are being trained "to do," rather than encouraged "to think"?

ImMEDIAtes represent the youngest generation discussed in this book and are the adolescent-plus generation who range in age from the teen years to early twenties. Your best pal is your phone—so much so that you panic if you are separated from your phone even briefly. It knows more about you than your parents or your friends. You keep it so close to your side that you even sleep with it. But oddly enough, you rarely use it as a phone; instead you use it for texting and logging on to social media outlets for immediate access to answers and to massive networks of people.

> As an ImMEDIAte, your attachment to your personal communication device is as integral to your being as eating and breathing.

A recent report found that one in three college students considers being able to connect to the Internet as important as fundamental resources like air, water, and shelter.[1] If this constant dependence on technology sounds like an addiction, in some instances, it just may be, says Dr. Nora Volkow, director of the National Institute on Drug Abuse. Dr. Volkow explains that just the emotional surge experienced when you receive an unexpected text fires up the dopamine cells in the brain. Dopamine is a neurotransmitter positively associated with pleasure, but it also plays a role in reinforcing addictive behaviors. In essence, you get high just thinking about who is texting you or what the message might be.

As an Immediate, you interact primarily through media; it is the main channel for how you initiate, keep, and terminate relationships. It is how you network with your friends, teachers, parents, and most everyone who wants to be in touch with you at all times of the day and night. Even passing between classes, you would rather text a friend than meet up to have a two-minute face-to-face conversation. Immediates thrive on sharing and knowing where "friends" are at any point in time and what their views are on any and every topic—ranging from the most trivial to the tragic to the triumphant. In fact, your connections are not limited by proximity or geographic boundaries. Your connections are far and wide—even continents away.

Technology is rewiring your brain daily so that you are becoming addicted to being distracted. One report showed that one in five college students say they are interrupted six times or more every hour when doing their homework—an average of at least once every ten minutes.[2] What's more, the same report noted that one in ten students said they lose count how many times they are interrupted while they are trying to focus on a project.

Boost your brainpower: Take your own tally of how often you are interrupted when doing your next project.

Certain habits are taking a toll on development of critical reasoning skills and innovative thinking in Immediates. Social networking and information overload may be major thieves stealing your brain performance. **Technological progress is obstructing individual creativity and failing to inspire your generation's capacity to think for yourselves.** The detrimental effects of technology on your generation's brain prowess are happening worldwide and are issues for concern. You can change your habits and alter your path to one of innovation, weighed reasoning, and deeper thinking by knowing when and when not to let your technology rule your thinking.

Boost your brainpower: Take on the challenge of not allowing yourself to be constantly interrupted and see how much faster you get your homework done or how much better you perform on a school or work-related assignment.

With instant access to the Internet through laptops, iPads, and cell phones, Immediates always have massive amounts of information instantly available at their fingertips. By posting and updating information through your social media channels, you rapidly influence available knowledge. However, there is a downside. Beware of your media's drawbacks. **You may be developing a blind trust in technology, and a large percentage of the information you are bombarded with is inaccurate, incomplete, and unqualified by valid facts.** You are perhaps unknowingly letting computers do the bulk of your thinking. You habitually and deftly retrieve information and rapidly recall an amazing quantity of facts and details from topics that interest you and even from topics that do not. As an Immediate, you are building a brain that knows how to store and retrieve facts with a speed that is hard to match or beat.

Though your generation is scoring perfect or near perfect scores on the SAT, ACT, GRE, MCAT, LSAT, and GMAT, many of you who are making the highest scores on entrance exams and achieve the highest grades in your classes are all too often failing to harness your full brain potential. **Top marks in school and on exams do not predict who will make the best doctor, teacher, parent, innovator, scientist, lawyer, business executive, or any chosen career expert.**

Why is this the case? **Your intense search for the immediate, correct answer does not necessarily lead to expanding curiosity and enhanced capacity to solve the complexity of problems that may plague your generation for the next decades.** In other words, the emphasis on speed of information access may be weakening your brain fitness at a time when you should be strengthening your brain's strategic and deeper thinking capacity.

And still, there are other Immediates who may have low grades or low scores on IQ or SAT tests. These tests are rigid, though rigorous, measures of fact-based learning and often incorrectly and detrimentally ascertain an Immediate's potential. **The momentous principle to remember is that performance on these structured tests does not define your potential.** These tests do not evaluate the entire range of fluid thinking that comes from deeper processing and practical problem solving that awaits you if you work daily to unlock your full potential.

A portion of the blame can be directed at how the education system is focused on test performance rather than training students how to generate new ideas; however, **a large degree of responsibility is on you** and the way you depend on quick access to knowledge as the way to learn. Current education practices are not elevating your brain health fitness and perhaps are even contributing to its decline. The causes of the downward trend in cognitive fitness of reasoning and critical thinking are multifactorial, but many are pointing not only to the continual distractions you actively seek, but also to the overemphasis on high-stakes standardized testing and teaching to the test.

> Immediates taught in a mechanistic, rote style of stuffing away facts for a test will build very different brains than those trained to abstract, synthesize, and connect meaning to their own world and other vast knowledge sources.

Sir Ken Robinson, in his updated edition of *Out of Our Minds: Learning to be Creative,* warns that we are not educating youth to take their place in the economies of the twenty-first century.[3] The current system of education was designed for a different age, namely the Industrial Revolution, where public education did not exist and youth had minimal access to information. What motivated students years ago to go to school may no longer work today. In the name of education, schools are slowly diminishing student capacities to excel in divergent thinking on tasks such as coming up with as many ways as possible to interpret a question.

For years parents and educators have preached, "The more you know, the better." The system has been building, training, and rewarding Immediates for spouting off numerous facts, leading you to value the rote memorization of data, a skill that stymies creativity. **One lesson to embrace now and throughout your life is: the more you learn, the more you will be humbled by how little you know and have yet to learn.**

Think about thinking—not knowing. Brain science is revealing that access to massive amounts of information is not making any of us smarter, regardless of age.[4] The Immediate generation is living in an era when being exposed to too much data and vast numbers of choices is your daily bread. But what if this voluminous cafeteria of options is hindering your brain's ability to adequately weigh the pros and cons to make healthy choices? Because your brain's frontal lobe is developing this lifelong powerful capacity during your current life stage, too many choices are actually stalling the development of decision making in your brain.

Just imagine when you were first learning to talk. Instead of learning your first words by being exposed to one, maybe two languages, imagine being exposed to ten languages all at once and simultaneously learning to talk. That enormous exposure to many diverse languages would make learning to talk harder, not easier. Similarly, information overload is crippling your development in making wise choices.

Another obstacle to achieving your brain potential is a falsely held belief that being exposed to more of the adult world sooner is making you grow up faster. Physically, you look more grown up earlier, but the brain's frontal lobe maturation is not happening faster. In fact, the opposite may be

> Less is more for brain development of sound decision making.

happening. All of this no-holds-barred access is making the Immediate generation mature slower. One key reason for this stalled development is that the immense number of opportunities stalls and overwhelms your choice making. In essence, your Immediate brain is almost frozen by the many choices in front of you.

So how do you handle it? Oftentimes you do not make a choice because the rapidly changing and yet immature stage of frontal lobe development makes decision making very undependable. **Your brain's maturation is at a vulnerable developmental crossroad, when rational judgment is unfolding and dangerous choices are real options.** You are better equipped to make sound choices when faced with one or two alternatives—such as places to meet your friends, colleges to apply, or even where to eat.

As an Immediate, you will learn sound judgment and weighed decision making by seeking advice from adults whom you trust—your parents, teachers or mentors. You will be often faced with some of the toughest life issues at an early age that necessitate even more guidance than when you were younger and did not have such risky options at your doorstep. The more you seek wise counsel, the more you will help yourself maximize the brain potential of your frontal lobe development.

There is obviously a delicate balance between being allowed to make the majority of your own decisions versus controlling how those decisions and judgments are made. If there is too much adult control, you will be at greater risk for not developing adult-level sound decision making. *If you do not have safe and stable boundaries, you may find yourself in deep trouble because you lack the skills to reason your way back to healthy choices.* Practicing frontal lobe skills and pushing the boundaries of decision making, planning, and having to suffer the consequences—however grave—seem to be prerequisites for adequate frontal lobe development.

Parents and guardians: do not act as your Immediates' frontal lobe in every instance nor remove consequences—this will stall your Immediates' cognitive development.

Whereas you are at a vulnerable life stage, you are also at a very creative stage in your life. Rote memorization of information stifles your desire to learn and become an innovator. Moreover, information is turning over so quickly, much of it at your fingertips through the Internet, that you fail to see the point in learning something for a test, knowing you'll forget the information shortly afterward. You are more motivated to create new ideas than learn facts that you can readily access. As an Immediate, your brain is primed to be challenged to develop deep-thinking capacity in order to expand frontal lobe function and to maximize intellectual capital. You need to take this challenge seriously because it matters now and for the rest of your life.

Never has our country been more worried about the future brain health of the young, particularly the way your minds are developing (or perhaps not developing). Alarms are sounding across the nation and around the world about the failure to maximize the brainpower of your generation. **As an Immediate, do not let the system limit your potential. You have control over your brain destiny, but it takes persistence and dedication.** Do not let circumstances limit your potential.

Take Philip, a senior in high school, whose teachers and parents were concerned about his lackluster school performance, which had become increasingly mediocre over the past two to three years. They were worried that his performance would end up hurting his chances to get into a good college. His parents reported that he read and researched on the Internet and worked on assignments for hours, but did not know how to translate all of those efforts into completed course projects. Philip's teachers suggested to his parents that he likely had attention deficit/hyperactivity disorder (ADHD). He didn't sit still for long, had been labeled lazy, and often failed to turn in homework assignments. Though he was producing excellent work in some classes, he was failing two others.

Philip's performance on all three core frontal lobe domains of strategic attention, integrated reasoning, and innovation were significantly below what he should be capable of given his high intelligence. He had not learned how to maximize his intellectual brain worth. His brain was quickly overwhelmed by the amount of information he was trying to absorb and he shut down, lost confidence, and no longer put forth effort. He was having significant difficulty in his history classes because he had to memorize a vast number of dates and places. He said, "I am all about the present and the future. Besides, I can look up all the old dates if I need to know them."

With regard to integrated reasoning, Philip was particularly deficient at being able to use knowledge to create new ideas. He had not learned to engage his advanced reasoning capacity and was stuck at a literal level in his ability to understand and absorb content. He was unable to combine concepts and synthesize meanings to advance his higher-order thinking ability.

Lastly, Philip's innovative performance was stilted as he could only squeeze out one or two ideas—not pushing himself to generate more—and thought that was sufficient.

Do you relate to Philip as a powerful representative of your Immediate generation? Do you feel like you are failing to reach your full intellectual potential? Philip is highly intelligent but is not adequately developing frontal lobe strategies to engage in dynamic thinking to prepare for the future. He needs to become adept at using knowledge to enhance his creativity. Right now Philip is experiencing information overload, and his ability to think for himself is stalled, thwarting his capacity to generate innovative ideas. He does not think of himself as being smart and is losing his confidence as a learner. The system is failing to inspire his brain-building curiosity.

According to *Lost in Transition: The Dark Side of Emerging Adulthood* by Christian Smith[5] adolescents are now:

- slower to emerge into adulthood.
- taking longer to graduate from college, if they graduate at all.
- depending on their parents longer.
- marrying later.
- struggling to find jobs.
- failing to work at stable jobs for any extended length.

All of these responsibilities are mediated by frontal lobe brainpower. Immediates as a group are struggling because their significant influencers are failing them, and Immediates themselves are struggling to properly engage their strategic thinking during a critical stage of development, **thus inadequately developing mature frontal lobe capacity. This does not have to be your story,** if you take steps now. You can become a brain fitness buff by establishing brain habits that strengthen your fluid intelligence skills. These are the skills that are necessary to flexibly use your mental resources to:

- identify problems that need to be solved.
- envision a major goal to achieve and determine the steps to get there.
- sort out what is enhancing and what is blocking forward progress.

- figure options to get out of life ruts.
- become more than completers of tasks.
- have confidence to innovate new approaches.

As an Immediate, be inspired by knowing that you are at a life stage where you have immense potential for brain expansion, if you take advantage of it. The sooner, the better. The brain undergoes more changes during these years from adolescence until midtwenties than in any other time except for the first two months of life. The changes can be seen dramatically in the frontal lobe, the area responsible for planning, reasoning, decision making, and other high-level cognitive functions. The Immediate years are a critical time for developing the fundamentally necessary strategic-thinking skills to guide you for a lifetime, because your brain's frontal lobe is primed to undergo rapid development. The caveat is that it now appears that this higher-level cognitive capacity does not unfold on its own but requires proper stimulation, exposure, and training to fully develop. Working to improve strategic thinking skills lays the foundation for the advanced reasoning that should be continually refined in complexity and maturity throughout adulthood.

Frontal Lobe Brainpower of Immediates

Frontal brain networks undergo dramatic expansion and remodeling during the Immediate stage of life. Education is neglecting the fourth "R" of education—reading, 'riting, 'rithmetic, and now *reasoning*.

Embrace this stage with all the gusto you can muster. As an Immediate, you are at a life stage where your brain is particularly primed to acquire the abilities that comprise the foundation of integrated reasoning (see chapter 5). You have probably heard your parents tell you the age when you learned to walk, talk, and read, because deeply ingrained developmental milestones exist for these skills. But there is controversy over whether or not critical reasoning skills can be taught, acquired, and applied across a wide variety of contexts.

Research has shown that some degree of reasoning may evolve on its own with the maturation of the frontal lobe, given proper environmental opportunities.[6] However, it appears that reasoning training may be necessary now more than ever since the vast majority of youth (upward of 75 percent) are failing to develop advanced reasoning even in the best environments. One key question is: Can individuals be taught how to *think about thinking* in such a way that it will provide a road map of strategic learning that could transfer across course content areas? Or is it a skill that if you have difficulty, you will always struggle with being a strategic and deep thinker much as if you were dyslexic and would struggle with reading? In this case, it is never too early or too late to develop strategic and innovative thinking skills. Your brain will be energized when you take them on, especially during the Immediate years.

Janet is an extraordinarily bright Immediate, a tenth grader, but the tragic news is that she is suffering immensely and not able to maximize her intellectual potential. She is driven to make high grades in every class. She stays up until the wee hours of the night overcompensating to overlearn everything so she can ace her tests. She has developed a very poor self-image and has been told that she is lazy, unmotivated, and stupid compared to others. She exhibits signs of anxiety and depression and is developing sleep problems.

Janet's performance on the core frontal lobe measures revealed extremely low strategic attention performance. Not only does she not block out information that does not need to be learned, she adds extraneous information. She is showing a pattern of **faulty gatekeepers** (see chapter 4). She is trying to remember everything and lets the gates open too wide so that irrelevant information, even information that was never presented, intrudes on her learning and thinking. She's a miserable memorizer, but that's how she is being judged as smart or not.

Her frontal lobe cognitive strength shone through in her advanced capacity to creatively combine separate ideas into synthesized meanings, indicating a high level of performance on integrated reasoning. Janet's ability to generate a number of innovative ideas, however, was very limited and narrow compared to what would be expected based on her integrated reasoning capacity. Her classroom training and testing was focused on getting the correct answer—that approach was clearly stifling her creative capacity to generate novel ideas. She was trying to please her parents and her teachers, but she was completely bored by the monotony of school, and all the facts she had to learn verbatim were causing her to **lose confidence in her own thinking.** The distressing paradox is that Janet is a creative thinker, not a rote, robotic learner. She is not being challenged to expand and stretch her fluid intelligence potential. In fact, just the opposite is happening, and she is paying the price.

In this period of information overload and constant distraction, as an Immediate, you will need to think more strategically about how to extract deeper meanings from complex information, apply them to your life issues, and develop study habits that focus on advanced reasoning and generating new ideas from what you are learning. **When you feel mentally stifled or when your brain feels frozen, it may be that you are approaching learning as a masterful memorizer.** Consider whether or not you're trying to superficially scan too much information with not enough time, rather than taking time to process smaller chunks of information more deeply and creatively.

You have the power to take control of how to ask new questions, not just try to answer a finite issue. Sure, education needs to be revamped to inspire your immense advanced reasoning and innovative thinking capacity. But you can be the instigator or agent of change by becoming part of the paradigm shift in showing how you transform rote facts into futuristic ideas. Surprise your teacher and your parents. Surprise your boss and mentors. Surprise yourself with your ability to stretch the boundaries of your imagination.

If properly enlisted, the brain can be mobilized to catapult you to a new level of thinking, of creating, helping to develop the prerequisite smarts and creativity to build a productive life. During the Immediate years, take advantage of:

- One of the richest epochs of brain modifiability
- The primed capacity of the human mind to think critically, which can be fine-tuned during adolescence and the twenties
- The emanating ability to synthesize meaning from complex information
- The brain fuel that arises from motivation and enables you to be innovative and think in novel ways

Brain Health Fitness

To think that you are building an unhealthy brain, unfit to solve the complexities of your early adulthood and beyond, is startling. Whatever the factors, as an Immediate you may not be developing the three core frontal lobe skills—strategic attention, integrated reasoning, and innovation—at the same rate and level as previous generations at your age. Some of the problems are outlined below:

Strategic attention: the ability to filter and focus on vast information (defined in chapter 4).

You are continually attending to everything at all times due to hypervigilance to your social media alerts. The ability to suppress unwanted information is a developmental cognitive process that should improve during the Immediate life stage if properly exercised. Blocking information is an active cognitive process, and when it works, the brain shows increased activation in the frontal lobe combined with reduced activation in medial temporal lobe regions.

Often you are asking your brain to work harder to focus because it has to actively block out extraneous background noise and switch back and forth between constant interruptions, hindering its efficiency. As a result, your brain is developing a faulty and inadequate filtering system. My team and I are currently looking into what percentage of Immediates has significant difficulty with strategic attention, but we estimate it to be upward of 75 percent. This could explain why large numbers of your generation are being diagnosed with attention deficit/hyperactivity disorder.

As a general rule, you are not building or strengthening your ability to sift through information and decide what's important versus unimportant. You might counter that it's because you do not have the knowledge base to separate the wheat from the chaff, but this deficiency is present even when knowledge is within your expertise.

Boost your brainpower: See if you have difficulty blocking what is irrelevant when you read something. Can you mark through the less important information, omitting at least 50 percent or more? Just imagine how hard it is to learn when every statement on the page seems to be of equal importance.

Thirty-five percent of Immediates drop out of school because of academic challenges, and many of you feel you do not want to, nor can absorb, all you're being asked to learn.[7] This push to memorize what can readily be looked up may be squelching your brain curiosity; there is too much low-level information for the brain to learn or to be inspired to innovate.

Think about this: you are keeping your brain in a continual state of vigilance to distraction. As a result, your brain stays too overtaxed and overwhelmed to promote deeper-level thinking and learning. **Left in this state of mind, you will be a robotic, unthinking consumer of information instead of a dynamic, flexible, creative thinker prepared to launch into a productive adulthood.**

Without the gating mechanism to filter unnecessary information out, the heavy load of information, which the mind is trying to handle, is too much.

Integrated reasoning: the ability to synthesize disparate pieces of information to form novel ideas, solutions, and directions (described in chapter 5).

New evidence indicates that the ability to synthesize meaning through integrated reasoning is declining in normally developing Immediates despite strong recall of the facts and details.[8] The studies reveal a stall in development of this capacity with as many as 85 percent failing to reach expected criteria.[9–10] Although our brains are intricately designed to be great synthesizers, the skill of integrated reasoning must be acquired. Through research at the Center for BrainHealth, my team and I have now evaluated integrated reasoning in Immediates across all socioeconomic levels.[11] At benchmark testing, the news is bleak. The Immediates we have assessed show dramatic deficiencies in the ability to think on their own and create multiple abstract answers to issues. We are actively searching for ways to empower youth, to transform classrooms into a rich context of inspired brain building, and to solve this crisis through cutting-edge research and training protocols. You will see how later in this chapter.

Innovation: the ability to solve new problems encountered; the ability to design and offer novel ideas and new directions at work or in academic learning (chapter 6).

Okay, this is not good news. You, at this young Immediate age, are already manifesting deterioration in your innovative thinking compared to what you could do even five years back. A longitudinal study indicated that divergent thinking (the ability to see multiple sides of issues or to generate large numbers of interpretations) peaks in primary school and gradually diminishes through early adolescence.[12] It's alarming that higher-level abilities are declining even at your young age, since we know that the immense power of the frontal lobe is just beginning to take off during this life stage.

How could the frontal lobe capacity of Immediates already be in a state of decay—going backward—before its time? A major contributing factor is that in the current education system, **Immediates are being trained to think of each question, first as if it had only one answer, and second, that the answer will never change.** This is a tragedy for the goal of increasing your human cognitive potential because the current situation is restricting the scope of your fluid intelligence.

> In essence, your brain may be losing capacity despite being in a life stage where brain potential should be increasing.

Enhancing Immediates' Brain Potential: Getting SMARTer

In this world, where information is being turned over at lightning speed, brain training practices of teaching what to learn will build out-of-date brains. Think about how you are trained to take college entrance exams. Since the questions are constantly changing, it is more about a strategy of test taking and less about the answers.

The extensive growth of the brain during the teen-plus years makes this an optimal time to train reasoning and higher-order creative thinking skills. One way to train higher-order creative thinking skills is through a unique and scientifically proven program called Strategic Memory Advanced Reasoning Training, or SMART. Developed at the Center for BrainHealth, SMART is based on cognitive neuroscience principles of how to best exercise the rapidly developing frontal brain networks.[13] SMART teaches Immediates to improve brain efficiency through organization, synthesis, abstraction, and constructing unique and novel ideas and approaches to doing things. Brain science has shown that constructing novel, generalized meanings is how the brain best learns. The SMART program teaches Immediates *how* to strategically think rather than *what* to learn.

SMART teaches Immediates techniques for deeper processing of information and critical innovative thinking, enabling longer-lasting understanding, better grasping of generalized significance, and inspired novel and creative applications of knowledge. The focus is on the three core frontal lobe functions, including strategic thinking, integration, and innovation.

- **Strategic attention:** Immediates learn how to focus with laser precision on the tasks and decisions that matter.
- **Integration:** Immediates learn to synthesize ideas from complex information across diverse multimedia and engage in futuristic thinking.
- **Innovation:** Through the SMART program, Immediates learn to construct insightful interpretations, imagine potential problems, identify multiple solutions, create novel directions, and view issues from diverse perspectives.

Helping students think SMARTer

Immediates become engaged in classroom discussions as they are challenged to think strategically and respond to readings with fresh, self-generated ideas. When you push yourself to think about content beyond the literal facts, you will glean insightful meanings and new applications to lessons. Moreover, as you begin to construct novel generalized meanings in one class, research at the Center for BrainHealth reveals that you can transfer this strategic approach across contexts such as science, history, math, and reading. When you continually challenge yourself to synthesize and create your own meanings, you brain performance skyrockets. Yes, you can rewire your brain at this young age.

My research shows:

- You will experience gains across core content areas, such as social studies, reading, math, and science, when you apply

generalized strategies to absorb and transform meaning (see chapter 5).
• Your love of learning will be reignited when you are encouraged to think and engage in lively interactions beyond answering specific questions with a single correct answer.

Research also discovered that Immediates at all levels of proficiencies showed gains—from the lowest performing to those with the most potential:

• 78 percent of the lowest-performing Immediates showed improvement after SMART.
• High-potential Immediates (like Philip and Janet) showed gains to superior range of advanced reasoning.
• Results showed dramatic gains in integration reasoning as well as generalization to other untrained areas.
• Statewide assessment scores for math, science, reading, and social studies show doubling of commended performance (the highest performance possible) after SMART (see graph below).
• Hispanic and African-American students demonstrate gains in reasoning ability similar to Caucasian students.
• All income levels make comparable gains in reasoning ability after SMART.

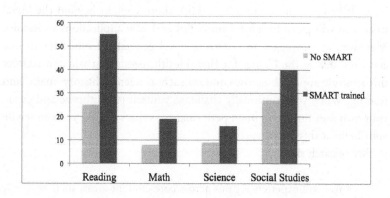

Building the core frontal lobe capacities to acquire new knowledge will be one of the most powerful brain training regimens you can adopt for life. It will help you apply old knowledge in novel contexts, chart new and insightful directions, specify unidentified problems and approaches, flexibly extract meaning from various sources, construct new abstract ideas, and cultivate futuristic thinking. **Brain science has shown that constructing novel, generalized meanings is how the brain best learns.** You will be ready for a futuristic workplace—one that does not even exist today.

Boost your brainpower: Try this when you are studying for your classes. Read the assignment and concoct your own abstract meanings in your notes. You will enhance your independent thinking capacity and also reinforce your ability to learn and apply the fundamental facts to boot.

By practicing the habits of formulating generalized principles and meanings, you will look forward to classroom discussions. Your brain is invigorated when you challenge it to compose new ideas and reasoning instead of regurgitating precise facts. **Take the strategic thinking challenge to see if you can transform yourself into an enthusiastic learner as you interpret content in new ways.**

Basic fact retrieval is boring when contrasted with the soaring pleasure of creating new knowledge. Creating makes learning worth it.

Real-Life Improvements in Advanced Reasoning

Below is a true story that represents the life-changing effects that are possible when the pivotal window of Immediate brain development is advantageously engaged.

Thirteen-year-old Cole had always been successful in school, making mostly As. In fact, he was in the talented and gifted classes through seventh

grade. In middle school everything began to decline—his school performance, his self-confidence, and his peer relationships. His tests and class
project grades began to drop, some even to failing level. His parents were
repeatedly talking to his teachers to try to get at the root of his learning
decline. They took him out of public school and put him in a private school
to see if smaller classes would help. Cole continued to fall behind even more
and began to think of himself as a poor student. He was completely overwhelmed by every assignment and felt he could never master the massive
amounts of information he was trying to learn.

At pretesting, Cole's Test of Strategic Learning revealed that he was at-
tempting to learn everything verbatim. After ten sessions of brain training he learned how to engage in top-down processing (such as identifying
themes, abstracting ideas, and giving interpretations) instead of bottom-up
learning (isolated facts). At post-testing, Cole was able to combine separate
concepts into abstracted, self-created ideas. He was able to more quickly
process the content from academic assignments. He showed a dramatic increase in ability to generate rich interpretations from readings. Moreover,
his ability to remember the basic facts significantly improved.

Cole, his parents, and his teachers observed the benefits of the training.
His study time went from six hours per assignment to about forty-five minutes when he began to think about and learn bigger ideas first (top-down
processing), rather than memorize isolated facts. Cole was no longer failing
and instead was at the top of his class in most courses.

"After training, I felt so much smarter—like I knew exactly how to learn
and think for myself. I felt inspired at school when I stopped trying to
remember everything exactly as it was printed. I am much more creative."

"After the training, Cole became a confident and efficient learner," his
father Joe said. "His conversations even showed more depth of thinking.
He now feels there is no goal he cannot achieve and has for the first time set
high expectations for his future."

Dramatic progress can be made by enlisting your frontal lobe to maximize
your brain potential. By engaging the frontal lobe networks to think strategically, you will be transformed into innovative and inspirational leaders.

Parents: How do you help your Immediate?

A time of extraordinary promise and vulnerability, this critical life stage merits larger-than-life attention from parents, brain scientists, educators, policy makers, and economists. Encouraging brain health fitness will set the stage for a productive life.

- It is important to teach Immediates to conceive of their own unique interpretations of movies; political discussions; local, national, and worldwide tragedies; unsettling school issues; bullying situations; or interpreting their own art creations to stimulate their frontal lobe brain function.
- Encourage them to be problem finders and designers of solutions for the context above or others that arise daily, using their new knowledge.
- Engage Immediates in discussions and reward reflection and imaginative thought grounded in reality instead of just listing the facts.
  * Ask your teenager to give you a "message" from a movie rather than a long-winded retell.
  * Have them interpret the lyrics of their favorite song from positive and negative perspectives.
- Encourage curiosity and train selective attention—the ability to focus on one object, voice, or thought—and to ignore or suppress nonattended or competing inputs.
  * Have them develop their own experiment to study uninterrupted, in a quiet environment on one course, versus studying with normal interruptions as usual on another course. Have them evaluate their own performances with their own rating scales as well as by their class grades.
- Inspire creativity and push for a multitude of answers to a question or problem versus seeking the "right" answer.
  * Have them imagine as many new phone apps as possible that would help to make usable reminders of things to do.
  * Share an ethical dilemma you are dealing with and have them advise you with as many good responses as pos-

sible, such as someone at work is sneaking out early
continually at a cost to coworkers.
* Watch their favorite television show and share in an
exchange about different take-home messages for the
different characters.

Brainomics of the Immediates

The worst-case scenario for brainomics is dramatically unfolding in the Immediate generation. Lifetime habits are being set in motion at this pivotal development stage that will have lasting ramifications on later economic productivity and health of individuals. I first conceived the notion of brainomics to capture the consequential relationship between educational achievement and economic well-being in the teen generation. Though this relationship may be most vividly portrayed in this generation, I subsequently realized that it applies to all stages of life.

It is becoming more apparent that the ability of any developed country to maintain a competitive edge in the global economy will depend on the competency of reasoning and critical thinking skills of your generation—the Immediates. Yet the current stats on achievement of your age group reflected on cognitive tests are staggeringly bleak:

• Reasoning, creative innovation, and critical thinking skill are stagnating in the United States.
• In a recent Programme for International Assessment (PISA) study, the United States ranked seventeenth out of twenty-seven participating developed countries in critical thinking and reasoning.[14]
• The United States ranked twenty-third out of twenty-seven in math, and seventeenth out of twenty-seven in science, as compared to other developed countries.
• More American teens are dropping out of high school than at any time in history. It is estimated that one teen drops out every twenty-six seconds, resulting in an average one million dropouts each year.
• Almost one-third of all public high school students fail to

graduate from high school with their class according to John Bridgeland, president and CEO of Civic Enterprises, whose research, *The Silent Epidemic: Perspectives of High School Dropouts,* was published in 2006.[15]

- Roughly two-thirds of U.S. teens, including those who graduate from high school, are unprepared for college work.
- Educators, public policy experts, and cognitive neuroscientists recognize the pervasive crisis of adolescents failing to thrive academically and personally as they transition from secondary and tertiary schools to real life but are unsure of the solutions to this dilemma.

Investing in the creative cognitive capital of your generation now can have a significant positive force on major economic growth, particularly in the long haul. **Enhancing brainpower will have an exponential benefit on economic growth. Our human cognitive capital is our greatest natural resource and yet we are letting it lay barren. How we teach students to become innovative, independent thinkers and train young professionals will be the strongest predictor for our economic well-being for the short term and future.**

Economists show that cognitive gains, achieved through transformations in innovative educational practices, are closely associated with long-run economic growth potentials.[16] If the United States were to contend with the highest performing countries (such as Finland and Canada) in educational levels in math, reasoning, and science, the cost benefit would be an estimated $100 trillion dollars. As Eric Hanushek, from the Hoover Institution at Stanford University, and Ludger Woessmann, from the University of Munich's Ifo Institute for Economic Research, warned in their 2011 article that appeared in *Economic Policy,* we cannot underestimate the high economic cost of low educational attainment.[17]

The dynamic interaction between human brainpower and economic growth is a wake-up call to find viable ways for Immediates to achieve their optimal brain edge—our future demands it.

Hanushek and Woessmann clarify that improving education is not about throwing more money or more regulations at schools. In fact, there is *not* a significant relationship between more funding and better student outcomes. Instead, educational reform needs to be directed at enhancing deeper level thinking and innovative brainpower of Immediates—especially at this critical developmental stage for advanced reasoning.

As I said earlier, adolescence and early adulthood represents one of the most optimal yet vulnerable stages for cognitive development supporting imagination and innovation. Critical reasoning and strategic thinking skills typically undergo rapid expansion during adolescence and are refined in complexity and maturity throughout adulthood. The failure to engage Immediates in strategic thinking and innovative reasoning is happening across socioeconomic levels.

Every year that we fail to train strategic and inventive thinking and advanced reasoning in Immediates, we fail to invest in the future of our human cognitive capital. Elevating brainpower in impressionable Immediates is imperative to promoting independent and creative ways of living. Sparking your imagination can truly make a difference for all of us. You are the future of your family, your city, your state, and this nation.

What kind of brain do you want to build? Now is the prime time to start construction on and commitment to your foundational healthy brain habits. You will want to deeply mine your creative capital, the richest, more renewable natural resource you will ever own. This gain will be the difference in making the world a more sustainable place.

Know Brainers

1. Immediates are at greater risk for developing addiction than at any other stage in life.
2. The brainpower in Immediates requires different educational strategies than previous generations to prepare them to solve the complexities of future problems.
3. Creative thinking is already declining in Immediates, but proper training can reverse the downward spiral.
4. Frontal lobe capacities of strategic attention, integrated reasoning, and innovative thinking are core areas that

Immediates need to be strengthening during this critical stage of brain development.

5. Being allowed to make tough decisions as an Immediate is necessary for healthy frontal lobe development.

6. Thrill seeking is an important aspect of this developmental stage.

7. In every single aspect of your life, you are being exposed to more choices, which are contributing to a freeze or stall in your brain's development. Seek guidance from parents and mentors and face the consequences of your choices.

8. The Immediate brain is being neuroengineered to have faulty strategic attention due to the immense sensory overload from all the information competing for their attention.

CHAPTER 8

THE FINDERS, 25–35, AND THE SEEKERS, 36–45 YEARS OF AGE

In this chapter, I consider the current status and future potential to increase intellectual capacity in two groups—the Finders and Seekers. The Finders, ages twenty-five to thirty-five, are tasked with "finding" the answers and taking care of routines. The Seekers, ages thirty-six to forty-five, are "seeking" their place of value in the leadership ranks.

Questions relevant to Finders and Seekers include:

Once the frontal lobe is developed at age twenty-five to thirty, what mental activities improve your frontal lobe capacity?

Why does making top grades in college not readily translate to rapid advancement in the workplace?

How can you move from knowing how to quickly gather facts to knowing how to think creatively to invigorate your work satisfaction?

How does the work environment enhance or impede brain productivity?

How is Google changing the way we learn and remember?

Are you aware of when you are in trouble with information overload?

What are ways you can determine when to stay the course and when to be an agent of change in terms of healthy brain development?

Finders

Finders, those in their midtwenties to midthirties, crave and are addicted to finding. You are the point-and-click generation, accustomed to fulfilling your incessant need for information and answers to questions with a simple entry in a search bar.

Take Molly, a young, seemingly bright twenty-eight-year-old. She was at the top of her class throughout high school and college, and after graduation she landed a highly sought-after position as the assistant to the CEO of a company that makes eco-friendly products. For six years she received small incremental annual raises but was never given more responsibility.

> Finders have been trained to find the correct answers since grade school and are always searching for "the" right response.

She consistently recorded enormous amounts of information, writing everything down almost verbatim. She produced well-organized technical reports of meetings and set forth next steps based on exacting precise recommendations from attendees. None of these amazing feats of information management required self-generated, novel ideas.

When I met Molly she said she loved the company for which she worked but admitted that **she was bored and felt that her mind was stagnating in a *cut-and-paste* routine.** She felt appreciation from her boss but was limited in opportunity. She did not know how to move up, over, or out. Molly was not provided the opportunities she needed to neuroengineer her brain into one that could be innovative and solve the complex problems of the organization. She was quite literally stuck.

Think of the negative impact on **brainomics.** Imagine the kind of brain Molly was building in her robotic job responsibilities. After education is completed, the work environment is the major shaper and contributor to advancing further intellectual development. How was her brain being neuroengineered and how were the

> Searching for "the" answer does not maximize innovative brainpower.

limited work-related brain challenges impacting her bottom line now and for the future? Sure, she was in an all-knowing position, aware of and carefully documenting copious amounts of information related to the organization's pivotal projects. **What an economic loss to the company for which she worked by their failure to mentor and more thoughtfully advance her creative brainpower!**

Frontal Lobe Brainpower of Finders

As reported in the Immediates chapter, recent discoveries in brain science indicate that the brain undergoes dramatic changes beginning in the teenage years and continuing through the twenties up until the early thirties. I think it is imperative to repeat this powerful piece of brain news since you are at a life stage, i.e., a transformative window of brain development, where your brain is primed for maximizing its inherent capacity to advance high-level decision making, innovative thinking, and strategic reasoning for sound judgment needed for life. This cognitive stage is happening in parallel with dramatic remodeling in the complex frontal brain networks. This brain development requires an ability to move from collegiate book learning to on-the-job learning—where you are set on identifying new approaches to almost everything.

For many reasons, your frontal lobe brainpower is underdeveloped and may even be stalled. Vital time and effort are spent stimulating learning and cognitive development throughout college to build strong language, literacy, and historical perspectives on societal issues, basic scientific knowledge, and computational skills. However, brain science has shown that similar efforts are needed to build foundational strategic reasoning and innovative thinking skills.

Evidence of this cognitive brain stall is emerging more and more, which means it is even more critical to take full advantage of your brain potential now. Training these critical skills is paramount to prepare your brain for the future. When you were in school or college, you could lay the blame on the education system. Now it is up to you to crack open the door to achieve your highest brain performance. Will you look to be told what to do, or will you discover things that need to be done?

BrainHealth Physical in Finders

Strategic Attention

Strategic attention is the easiest cognitive function to enhance through practical applications in daily life. Finders almost instantly report back a substantial brain gain when they follow the Brain Powers of strategic attention: None (make time for down time), One (sequential tasking), and Two (identifying their elephants or big tasks). Reread chapter 3 to review how to incorporate these Brain Powers into your life. One element that has a critical impact on this function is technology.

I saw the negative effects of technology in two Finders I worked with recently. Both scored low on measures of strategic attention, and it was evident that instead of thoughtfully processing information, these two Finders showed their naiveté and demonstrated a great memory but an inability to strategically select and block information they were presented.

It is quite challenging for you to sort through all the information that inundates your daily life. Indeed, **your greatest deficit is being unable to block information from your attention. You try to process all the information presented instead of blocking 50 percent or more of what confronts you.** Because you, as a Finder, are accustomed to searching for and finding information, your knee-jerk reaction is to survey as much information as possible, typically through Internet searches. However, this detrimental habit bores your brain and overloads intellectual capacity.

> "The thing about technology is that it has made the world of information ever more dominant." —Jaron Lanier, computer scientist and author from UC Berkeley.

Integrated Reasoning

Evidence reveals that the more choices a person has, the less likely he is going to make a rational decision or even make a decision at all. The brain appears to get overwhelmed and even frozen with the burden of too much information.[1] This overload is preventing Finders from engaging in deeper, more strategic and innovative thinking.

Is it possible that more information is making us less smart—perhaps even stupider? There is not a straightforward answer. Roddy Roediger, a professor of psychology at Washington University in St. Louis, suggests that the gradual increase in IQ scores identified over the past hundred years may result from our information-rich environment.[2]

However, I warn that just because you are information rich and because we have seen a dramatic increase in IQ does not mean that fluid thinking has increased. Remember, IQ is an outdated, out-of-touch index of dynamic thinking (see chapter 1). Fluid thinking is exactly what you need to be smart in the future. This was incredibly evident in the two Finders I mentioned earlier. On measures of integrated reasoning in their BrainHealth Physical assessment, these Finders demonstrated a sophisticated vocabulary. However, the praise stopped there. They failed to exhibit dynamic and flexible thinking as manifested by inadequate utilization of the Brain Powers of Zooming (see chapter 5). They failed to zoom out from the details to derive bigger ideas and were unable to think of broader applications, instead being stuck in the literal information as presented. They simply skimmed the surface and retained superficial information instead of deeply processing what was presented.

> Finders are addicted to the need for speed.

You have grown up with modern, easily accessible technology. When people ask me if technology is good or bad for the brain, I say emphatically— "YES!" Inquisitive minds stare at me for a minute, but then the message is clear to them. Technology has been both good and bad for our brain development.

I would never go back to a time without technology. I can remember when I was working on my dissertation—it would take me two, sometimes three months to get access to certain research articles or books. Now, with technological advances, you have just about any article you want at your fingertips within minutes. This immediate access to information is a dream come true to a researcher and to most any business with rapidly changing schemas.

A recent study shows that Google has caused our whole memory systems to become revamped.[3] If we know we can look it up later, we don't recall information nearly as robustly as we would if we thought that we might not have access to the information online. In essence, individuals are able to remember the folder where the information was stored, but not the information. You no longer need to learn and remember facts—you just need to store data and know how to find it quickly.

At a recent speaking engagement, Jaron Lanier, a computer scientist guru who is best known for popularizing the term "virtual reality," asked his audience not to blog, text, or tweet while he was speaking. He was trying to stop the pervasive multitasking efforts that preclude people from being present and in the moment. His point of view: "The most important reason to stop multitasking so much isn't to make me feel respected, but to make you exist. If you listen first and write later, then whatever you write will have had time to filter through your brain, and you'll be in what you say. This is what makes you exist. **If you are only a reflector of information, are you really there?**"[4]

Finders have a laborious time taking notes in meetings beyond what is said verbatim. You report difficulty knowing how to conceive bigger ideas in real time. And often you fear that if you wait to write things down, you will forget the message. However, science shows that if you wait, you will

> Are you a reflector or a processor? Think about how you approach information.

process the information more deeply and integrate it through your own perceptions.[5] Doing so will change the hard-to-remember rote-meaning into something more personal and memorable, increasing your frontal lobe brainpower.

As a Finder, you have been rewarded for accuracy in how precisely you remember information as it was delivered, thus reinforcing a detrimental brain habit. As you learned in earlier chapters, **rote learning does not build the core frontal lobe skills that are indispensible for the fluid, dynamic intellect** necessary in a constantly changing world. For too many, the highest goal is accumulating information rather than generating new ways of thinking and innovative problem solving. However, effortful, thoughtful processing is key to healthy brain development. **Remember, complex thinking makes your brain healthier** (chapter 5). Pushing the limits of your brain function will not only be a boon to your personal brain development but will benefit the companies for which you work as well as the economy of our nation as a whole.

Innovation

As Finders, you have the opportunity to become visionaries more than any other generation, using social networking for brain gain rather than drain. But you have to guard against following the crowd blindly. In Jaron Lanier's book *You Are Not a Gadget: A Manifesto,* he claims that social-networking sites like Facebook and Twitter encourage shallow interactions.[6] He suggests that he hopes to revive the development of software to allow people to be creative. I suggest that this means technology has made the Finder generation, your generation, more robotic.

So, Finders, what does this mean for you? When I asked a group of Finders recently about when they felt their brain was/is or will be at peak performance, the majority answered that now is when they are maximizing their potential. While I am thrilled that these Finders did not think their best brain years were behind them, I was hoping they would realize that while they feel their brain is operating at a high level of performance, they still have an opportunity to go even higher. You have the ability to build your own brain by how you use it every day. Build a brain health plan to help you reach your brain fitness goals.

How are you going to increase your strategic attention, enhance your integrated reasoning, and increase your innovative capacity?

One Finder I recently worked with named Abby put the following brain health plan into place:

To improve her strategic attention:

- While on the phone, avoid checking emails or looking online and vice versa.
- Stop checking email and text messages at night before bed to limit overactive thought at night.

To enhance her integrated reasoning:

- Skim presented material once, but then go back through and spend time synthesizing the main takeaways and formulating big ideas from material.

To increase her innovative capacity:

- Mull over thoughts, contemplate ideas, and envision solutions instead of just immediately responding with the first thing that comes to mind.
- Carve out a small project rather than taking on more tasks, and develop visionary plans of action to achieve goals.

The possibilities are boundless now that you have the necessary strategies needed to boost your brainpower. The power is truly in your hands, or your head, to be exact, so take control and reach your maximum cognitive potential.

Brainomics of the Finders

Clearly, our general economy is suffering major current and future losses due to unrealized brain attainment. **How can you become prepared to solve minor and major national and world crises if your brain is primarily trained to always *find* an answer?** The answers you are striving to find probably do not even exist yet, and even if the answers were available, they would be too complicated to find in a point-and-click search in a source that is rarely validated. Finders need to move to the next stage of life where you have the responsibility to identify the core issues to be solved and generate the answers, rather than solely searching for data and explanations that already exist.

Indeed, Finders are failing to meet basic expectations as critical thinkers because you are not adequately harnessing and exploiting your own brain potential. You may have strong qualifications on paper, but if your intellectual capacity remains static, we will all suffer economic loss in the not too distant future.

Current leaders need to rethink how Finders' brains are being trained; it is up to those in charge of bringing on and cultivating new talent to capitalize on the potential brainpower of young adults. The potential is there but old ideas of productivity are repressing the developing fluid intelligence of the Finders by failing to

> Nurture versus nature: brainpower must be nurtured so that it's not a victim to the nature of our environment.

nurture their core frontal lobe functions of strategic attention, integrated reasoning, and innovation.

One place to enact change is in the workplace. Work environments provide the perfect life-laboratory where brainpower can be advanced or stymied in major ways. Corporate executives constantly approach me, saying, "We do not know how to integrate the smartest and brightest twenty- and thirtysomethings into our workplace. They are smart, have high GPAs and impressive résumés, but they cannot solve problems or even think what to do each day without being told exactly what to do. They need and want to be given a list of exactly what to achieve. They feel anxiety if they are left on their own to try to figure new ways to advance their work output and increase productivity."

One reason: the pervasive use of cubicles. Cubicles impede and are toxic to your brain health and stifle brain development. Ponder how the very nature of cubicles works against strategic attention and integrated reasoning. The whole concept was deliberately conjured up to spawn and foster more collaborative work habits that inspire innovation. Certainly, cubicles increase crosstalk among individuals considerably; however, the jury remains out as to whether this environmental design has been a boon or a disadvantage to innovative thinking. For sure, it has elevated cross-hearing where no such thing as a private conversation exists in a cubicle setting. Think of the cost to strategic attention—how hard the brain has to work to block out ambient conversation just to focus on the task at hand.

One Finder, Jeremy, told me that he did not know if he had ADHD or if he was just having a hard time blocking out all the stimulation from his surrounding coworkers in close cubicle spaces. He said that he suffered from migraines and wondered if the work environment was contributing to his brain drain. All of us know how hard it is to be productive when in pain. I advised him to talk to his boss about finding a quiet office space to work for short intervals, especially when it was a major project that demanded more focused attention. Jeremy reported back that this simple modification made a big difference in his brain energy and efficiency. His migraines dwindled as well.

I recently worked with Julie, a

> You are primed to develop your brain function and expand your innovative potential.

thirty-three-year-old marketing professional. At first glance, she seemed apathetic, disengaged, and disinterested in the day-to-day tasks of her job. She confessed, "I feel like I'm doing the same thing day in and day out; I rarely feel challenged and want more from my professional life." Indeed, her performance on her BrainHealth Physical revealed that she struggled with abstracting new ideas and rarely, if ever, applied innovative thinking to create solutions or different outcomes. She was stuck in concrete mode, searching for one clearly defined answer. She was not bridging meaning from what she was learning and observing with previous experience to generate new possibilities. Thus, her brain's generator, which was recycling information rather than combining separate ideas in creative ways, was easily bored and burned out.

Failing to engage in novel thinking and critical reasoning is detrimental to your brain and the advancement of thinking smarter—not harder. This failure is happening across all careers and all fields regardless of whether you are a high achiever or underachiever. Every year we fail to incite and arouse strategic novel thinking and advanced reasoning, we fail to invest in the future of our human cognitive capital.

Seekers

When I first developed my ideas for this chapter, I had lumped the ages from twenty-six to forty-five together as one generation. But as I began to talk to individuals in the *thirty*-six to forty-five age range, you told me that you were very different from the Finders. I stepped back and realized that even though there were many commonalities, there were striking differences between the two age groups.

Seekers are between a rock and a hard place in life. You are seeking to:

- Identify your place in society
- Figure out where you best fit in
- Determine where your growth potential resides

The Thinkers, or those between age forty-six and sixty-five, are your mentors and managers and are not readily turning over the reins to you in the foreseeable future. In fact, Thinkers seem to have balanced things out nicely. They can be the big-picture visionaries while Seekers, who report to them, can be the make-it-happen, detail-oriented group.

Couple this gray zone of leadership potential with the evidence that in the majority of countries the Seeker age group is the unhappiest. Why is this the case? The results have been interpreted to suggest that happiness dips in the Seeker years due to elevated stress, worry, and the complications of managing families—especially young teenagers.[7-8] Stress could be attributed to being stuck in jobs with no ability to see future growth.

Ted definitely feels stuck. He is a forty-two-year-old Seeker who came from out of town to find out if there was something more he could do to increase his mental productivity and leadership skills. He was:

- a chronic multitaskaholic,
- an information downloading junkie, and
- working long hours but getting less done.

He overcommitted himself, believing it would help him get an edge up on a promotion. The problem, as he described it, was that he reported to two people—both who were in the Thinker generation. Neither had any plans on retiring. The thing that frustrated him the most was that he felt his superiors had switched to an automatic pilot mode of operating and that he was carrying more of their load but getting paid much less. He felt he was a more strategic thinker, more expressive contributor in meetings, and more tuned into where the company should be going but was not.

I see Ted's situation in other people over and over again. He really is between a rock and a hard place because he does not know where to turn. He cannot go complaining to his boss.

Seekers: you are not climbing the corporate ladder at the same speed Thinkers did when they were in their thirties and forties. Twenty years ago, CEOs were commonly in their thirties and forties, but this is rarer now. Ted is looking for a new job where he can sprout his wings to lead. What a major loss it will be for his company and the leadership team. **The work environment is stalling his ability to increase his intellectual capital; brainomics is losing in this situation.**

Another Seeker, Shirley, is a different story. She is forty-one and has been promoted, currently serving as CEO of a national corporation with multiple businesses. However, she came to see me because she had some concerns. She felt:

- her high level performance declining.
- loss of motivation.
- excessively distracted.
- growing unhappiness with her work.

On her BrainHealth Physical, she exhibited inefficient strategic attention with her ability to apply strategies to focus and filter information getting worse with repeated trials. Her brain was quickly overwhelmed with information. Her integrated reasoning was extraordinarily low given the high complexity of the cognitive demands of her job. She excelled in innovation, being able to think fluidly and creatively with a multitude of interpretations. For Shirley, her intellect was being drained. She was definitely intelligent, but her brain energy was being depleted. One of the key areas I recommended that she improve was in prioritizing her efforts. She was trying to do it all, and giving everything the same level of attention. It's not possible for a brain to push wildly day in and day out. She did not know where her elephants were.

Finders and Seekers: here are some key ways to advance the core frontal lobe skills of strategic attention, integrated reasoning, and innovation:

1. **Strategic attention:** Use your elephant and rabbit to-do list pad from chapter 4 daily. Do not let your rabbits (low-priority tasks) turn into elephants (major objectives) so that you pay less attention to the assignments that will make the most difference daily.
   a. Practice sorting the essential from the trivial.
   b. Recognize which decisions require the greatest attention and which ones can be relegated to less effort.
   c. Train how to get the important decision right.

2. **Integrated reasoning:**
   a. Gain intellectual capital by mentoring others to rely on their executive decision making.
   b. Hone your skills in recognizing when your knowledge seeking is enhancing your deeper thinking and when it is freezing your mind from synthesizing higher-level ideas.

   c. Develop the brainpower of zoom deep and wide and
      combine your expanding expertise with newly emerg-
      ing ideas and criticisms.

3. **Innovation:**
   a. Engage in seeking new directions.
   b. Develop novel ideas.
   c. Reflect on where things may go in the future and how
      to stay ahead of the game.

Finders and Seekers are nearing a recipe for disaster because your environment is not building the type of brainpower that will ensure you are
leaders of tomorrow. Small changes can make all the difference and brain
growth can be impressive. It will take some flexibility and understanding on
the part of Thinkers and Knowers who manage you to make sure they are
harnessing the power of the next generations.

Know Brainers

1. Use technology to your advantage to manage
   information.
2. Strengthen your resolve to change your habits away
   from overloading and downloading data that is
   causing mind-freezing from the deluge of data.
3. Continue to challenge frontal lobe proficiency by
   blocking unimportant information, thereby letting the
   most important ideas take greater precedence.
4. Instead of searching to find the answer, spend time
   thoughtfully combining concepts to generate new
   ideas and solutions.
5. Consult only a limited number of information sources
   and think deeper about how the ideas can impact
   your team. (Make sure the source is credible.)
6. Mentor and be mentored to strengthen executive
   function skills to orchestrate new projects.
7. Advocate for yourself to receive training to
   make leadership decisions and take leadership

responsibilities to strengthen your frontal lobe networks.

8. Reflect on how your environment is inspiring or deflating your brain innovation at the end of each day.

9. Decide if you are afflicted by infomania (addicted to rapid communication responding) and if so, stop the rapid back-and-forth barrage that is taking its toll on your mental productivity.

10. Help develop a more efficient way to be focused and mentally present in meetings and on conference calls by making these oftentimes brain drains more inspiring and engaging for innovative exchange of ideas.

CHAPTER 9

THE THINKERS, 46–65 YEARS OF AGE

If you are between forty-six and sixty-five years of age, you are part of the Thinker generation, otherwise known as boomers. I labeled your group Thinkers as you tend to view yourself as thinking from a very unique and different viewpoint from the generations that came before. You did not necessarily go along with the thinking of the time, instead becoming an independent thinker who had the courage to take a stand counter to the popular views of the time. As a Thinker, you are part of one of the most optimistic generations and genuinely expect the economic opportunities and realities to improve with time. You are part of the healthiest and wealthiest generation, and you feel that with hard work you can change the world and your standard of living.

Questions relevant to Thinkers include:

Why do you worry about memory problems more than other diseases?
Are your best brain years behind you?
Are you working out your brain or burning it out with the daily mental challenges you take on?
What is robbing you of your brain value?
Can you keep from going backward in your brain performance levels?
How can you slow the rate of losses in your brain performance?
What can you do to make sure your intellectual reserves will last throughout retirement years?

Michael, a sixty-year-old Thinker and entrepreneur, explained when he felt that his brainpower and decision-making capacity were at their prime levels: "I think I am able to make better decisions now than ever before. For me, it's the difference between *learning* and *thinking*." He went on to say, "I may not learn as fast as I did when I was younger, but I can certainly think a whole lot better now. And even when I learn, I know how to do it better. I love to problem solve—the more complex the task, the higher the buzz I get from the challenge. The challenges I am now tackling would have eluded and overwhelmed me earlier in life."

Michael's sentiments vividly portray why I call the boomer generation the Thinkers. Thinkers have spent the majority of their adult lives relying on themselves to change and invent things and be entrepreneurs of ideas, companies, and solutions.

Maybe you've heard the story about the very self-important college freshman, or Immediate, seated next to a Thinker at a football game. The freshman had just explained to the Thinker why it was impossible for his older generation to understand his generation.

"You grew up in a different world, actually an almost primitive, unconnected one. My friends grew up with email, unstamped cards, texting, iPhones, iPad, iPods, cloud storage—even electric cars. We can be with our friends anytime, day or night, without being with them. We have wireless connections and high-speed computers that can think faster than you can blink."

When he paused to take a swig of beer, the Thinker took the opportunity to say, "You're right, son. We didn't have those things when we were young . . . so we INVENTED them. Now, you arrogant little tweeter, what are you doing for the next generation?"

Though not exactly a true story, it clearly illustrates my point that brainpower does not have a preference for a young brain. The latest challenge for Thinkers is to continuously maintain your highest level of performance as a CEO of your brain—Cognitive Entrepreneur Officer.

How Much Savings Are in the Thinkers' Intellectual Account?

Thinkers are a paradox. You are working nonstop—you stay connected at all hours to family and your professional life. You are addicted to working toward your goal: to retire as early as possible and maintain the comfortable lifestyle to which you have become accustomed.

Now, as a Thinker, you are faced with two dilemmas. The largest is that you may need to work longer since much of your financial nest egg has disappeared due to bad investments and a weakened global economy. The second is that you are anxious about losing your mental edge. **According to a recent MetLife study, your number one health concern is memory problems.**[1] In fact, for the first time in decades, you are more worried about memory loss—a potential harbinger of dementia—than you fear other health concerns such as heart disease, stroke, or diabetes. In one of my recent surveys of hundreds of Thinkers ages forty-six to sixty-five, 86 percent indicated that their memory was not as good as they would like and is often unreliable.

It is intriguing that memory is the key area Thinkers want to improve. **Memory grabs our attention because we experience glitches throughout our day** as vivid reminders that our mind is not a digital camera whose data can be quickly retrieved exactly as it happened with the push of a button. Are memory problems the big kahuna for Thinkers?

> We rarely stop to take inventory of all the things our brain remembered at the end of the day—instead we remember the few things that we forgot. Fascinating that we *remember* what we *forget*.

Build BrainHealth Fitness

When asked what kind of brains Thinkers would create for themselves if they could do some rewiring or what they wish their brains could do that they do not do now, I get responses like:

- Not deteriorate with time
- More memory capacity

- Ability to learn faster
- Learn with less effort
- Faster processing
- Faster search and recall
- Ability to turn off brain
- Improved analytical ability
- Photographic memory
- Manage stress effectively
- Remember names
- Not wander with thoughts
- More technically minded
- Exact replica of mine now, but faster
- Better retention

Thinkers are actively striving to test the limits of staying youthful longer—both physically and in terms of brainpower. The sixties are the new fifties—maybe even the new forties. Advertising is playing into this ego perspective. Infomercials scream, "If you buy this product, it will take five . . . ten . . . maybe fifteen years off your brain."

With age, it is natural to value youth in appearance. **Now this "stop aging" bias is carrying over to how you think about your brain.** There are valid reasons and scientific proof supporting the idea that as a Thinker, you believe your best brain years could be in the past. But don't put too much faith into this viewpoint—remember how fast I said brain facts are getting upended? Nonetheless, let's consider the evidence before I dispute it.

For example, look at the dismal current data indicating cognitive decline status in the figure below.

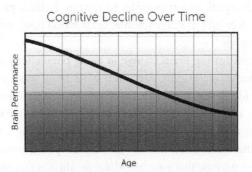

Cognitive Decline Over Time

Are Thinkers losing their intellectual capital at too rapid a
rate to avert the brain drain?

The downward spiral of cognitive decline resembles the Dow Jones average curves in periods of severe economic depression. If it were true, as a Thinker, you could be losing your intellectual capital at a faster rate than you can fend off! As measured, the peak years on select cognitive domains are around the late twenties to thirties. This young age of brain peak performance is precisely the period when the rich frontal lobe networks are reaching adult-level maturity.

Thinkers are aghast when I show the sharp decline in cognitive skills graph. Their moans are loudly audible. They are taken aback by the large body of research asserting that they are losing and becoming less efficient at engaging their brainpower.

A large number of studies from cognitive scientists, indeed, show that basic cognitive capacities begin to decline in our forties—earlier than the youngest members of the Thinker generation.[2-3] That such continual and unstoppable losses will accrue over time is *not* the type of news Thinkers will take sitting down—especially at such an early age—given that life expectancies are now reaching all-time highs. But these declines in cognitive performance are backed up with brain changes. Data from brain imaging studies support significant changes in brain structure and function in Thinkers and Knowers (those who are older than sixty-five) that could account for cognitive losses.[4-5] The frontal cortex, which is pivotal to higher-order thinking skills, shrinks and loses gray matter beginning at a relatively early adult age with a peak in our twenties to thirties. Indeed, prefrontal brain regions show decreases in brain volume, brain blood flow, and metabolism with increasing age.[6]

Studies investigating brain change in aging populations elegantly analyze large volumes of imaging data from MRI brain scans to try to offer explanations for different patterns of brain response. Some believe that Thinkers-plus may have to work their brains harder to achieve the same levels of performance as younger adults. People may use more mental effort, effectively using more "brain muscle" to maintain performance levels.

Researchers propose that younger adults use their brains more efficiently than older adults.[7] That is, they use less brain to accomplish the same task where older adults activate more regions. This shift is interpreted to indicate that perhaps the Thinkers' age group is restructuring how they use their brain networks to compensate for brain loss and cognitive decline. If this foreboding of cognitive loss were the whole story, why would I call a group whose brain is going down the drain the Thinkers?

I often ask those over fifty, **"Could you do what you are doing now, say, twenty years ago, even ten years ago?" Most, like Michael, honestly say they could not solve the complex issues they deal with today.** What would your answer be?

> Most leadership positions are held by Thinkers.

If such cognitive decline were the whole story, I would have dubbed this group the Relinquishers—giving up brain capital. Whereas the data is real, I believe the interpretation is defective and requires reconsideration and fuller examination.

I make my case by asking: "If you think brain performance in twenty- and thirtysomethings is at peak performance, have you spent much time with Immediates or Finders lately?" Please understand that I am not meaning to insult the younger generations who have immense potential; I just want us to rethink how we objectify intellectual brainpower. Society's conceptualization of what is smart is obsolete (chapter 1). I repeat this several times throughout the book so you'll take heed. IQ testing was established to make sure children with learning problems received the necessary intervention. Now the interpretation of IQ measurement has been blown out of proportion, its importance exaggerated, and the limitation of such testing has stifled how we envision the immense potential for the human mind. From my perspective, IQ testing may do more harm than good. As Sir Robinson states in his book *Out of Our Minds,* the popular notion of intellectual abilities has become dangerously narrow and other intellectual abilities are either ignored or underestimated. Using intelligence in a traditional sense may fail to capture the musings and innovations of the mind that get stronger with rich experiences and vast exposure to new complexities of life.

The discoveries about brain efficiency and the disparity profiles between age groups are in relatively early stages of exploration and need to be interpreted cautiously.[8] Indeed, in some studies more focal activation of the brain is interpreted as deficient and in others it is thought to indicate enhancement. For example, studies show that when adults move into early stages of dementia called mild cognitive impairment, their brain shows significant increases in activation.[9] When these individuals are compared to those who officially meet the criteria for dementia, the brains of the dementia group show considerably less activation when compared to either normal groups or those with mild cognitive impairment. The point is: arguments saying less brain activation is either better or worse depend largely on a number of individual factors.

> More brain activation may be either good or bad; the direction is not absolute.

A second major caveat to blindly accepting that Thinkers' brains are in a stage of decline rather than growth has to do with the data being collected largely from cross-sectional studies rather than longitudinal studies.[10] Whereas longitudinal studies follow the same individuals over time, cross-sectional studies compare age groups at one point in time. Imagine the mistakes we could make by comparing functionality across Immediates, Finders and Seekers, and Thinkers and Knowers in the year 2020. Given the fact that a brain is neuroengineered by how it is used at any age, you can just begin to imagine the immense differences and experiences that separate each generation.[11-13] Variables other than age contribute significantly to these differences. Consider how the use of technology for the present generation is building a very different brain compared to past generations.[14]

My BrainHealth team and others are upending the views of a brain in decline with age to recognize and build the fuller potential—the full frontal potential. Think about the amount and type of information to which a Thinker has in his or her knowledge repertoire versus what a Finder (twenty-six to thirty-five years of age) has to help them solve problems. Few would disagree that Finders have much less facts and experience stored up for expansive use. It is highly plausible that a higher data-rich brain could activate more brain regions as it has access to immense associations stored across brain areas.

Dr. Gene Cohen, the first chief of the Center on Aging at the National Institute of Mental Health and the first director of George Washington University's Center on Aging, Health & Humanities, once commented that an older brain may represent a more fully networked brain. As such, the Thinker's brain may actively integrate elements across diverse regions and between hemispheres to perform tasks. The Thinker's brain, with more elaborate content and widely distributed information brain networks than younger brains, could be a partial explanation for this. Thinkers engage more brain regions of activation than Immediates and Finders on select tasks.

With age, there is increased risk of adults having coexisting brain complications that can impair thinking that go beyond such aging changes as dementia. Researchers suspect that past studies on cognitive aging may have included participants who were in very early stages of dementia (where brain cell loss is rampant even though symptoms are not yet overt). Investigations must carefully screen out and exclude complicating brain conditions in adult populations. Otherwise the findings can lead to the wrong interpretations regarding the rich potential for brain gains even in advanced aging.

> A normal aging brain does not have to lose connections in the prefrontal cortex related to using knowledge and expertise.

Good News Is Growing

A team of scientists from Mount Sinai School of Medicine found that a certain type of brain connection responsible for engaging long-term knowledge and expertise was unaffected by normal aging.[15]

Take Betsy, a sixty-two-year-old president of a large investment firm. She is concerned about her mental decline and has been for the past eight years because Alzheimer's disease runs in her family. Betsy complains that her memory troubles her, and she is frustrated by the inordinate amount of time it takes her to absorb content. She reports that she has to read information five to six times just to get the key ideas.

Like many, Betsy is not the only one concerned; her colleagues and family have also brought her memory shortfalls to her attention. Betsy said, "I have always had problems. But now, my problems seem to be more blatant because of how much I have to read and the slowness I experience in gathering the most meaningful ideas. I feel at a disadvantage compared to my colleagues who can recall facts on a whim, but I still excel in my analytical ability." She asserts that she is "holding [her] own and still able to competently sort through the chaff and wheat to extract the core issues from meeting briefings at a level even better than five years ago." In fact, Betsy is recognized for her astuteness in culling out the critical issues.

So, what are the results of her BrainHealth Physical? On standardized cognitive testing, Betsy's memory is quite worrisome, falling three standard deviations below normal. Her speed of processing, concentration, and attention are all also significantly lower as compared to the norms.

In sharp contrast to these extremely low performances on lab tests, Betsy's performance on the three core frontal lobe domains of strategic attention (chapter 4), integrated reasoning (chapter 5), and innovation (chapter 6) were notably impressive. On the strategic attention measure, her profile was that of a Strong Strategic Attender—Quick Study (profiles described in chapter 4). She was able to immediately adopt an efficient strategy on the very first trial and continued to use it on the third trial. In fact, she was 100 percent efficient in recalling the high-priority items and completely blocking the low-priority items for trials one and three. **To employ this high-level filter-focus strategy so early and effectively was intriguing in the context of low memory performance.**

The strategic attention measure also evaluated her immediate memory span. Betsy's memory span was significantly lower than most Thinkers. Even still, she was above the majority, showing a perfect frontal lobe strategy for gating information from the beginning. That is, she exhibited a proficient ability to work around her memory problems at the highest level possible, spontaneously adopting a strategy to remember the most important items from the first try. Betsy's high level of strategic learning surprised even me, given her severe memory problems.

In regard to integrated reasoning, Betsy demonstrated an average ability to read new information and construct synthesized meanings by interpreting new information within the context of her rich repository of wealth of knowledge. In addition to stellar performance on strategic attention, Betsy also showed impressive innovation skills as reflected in generating a multitude of diverse high-level creative interpretations across three tasks. Her ability to answer specific probes on data retrieval was extremely low, again consistent with real memory problems.

Betsy's question to me was: "How can my horrible memory that I suffer day in and day out exist side by side with a high capacity to engage in the complex strategic thinking skills required in my job?" She continued, "I never fail to extract the best next steps in executive meetings; in fact, my team looks to me to come through on the big ideas. However, I do not keep up in remembering the point-by-point details of what had happened previously even close to others at our meetings. Still, I feel that I am at the height of my brain functionality in decision making."

I must confess I have not seen a person with such contrasting high functionality on our three core frontal lobe measures in the same context of such low memory functioning. My recommendations were surprisingly not directed toward increasing her memory span aside from trying to get someone to take high-level notes during meetings that she could review when thinking about next steps.

Rather, I gave Betsy specific strategies on how to strengthen her high aptitude for successfully linking disparate ideas for best next steps. I also suggested that she take time to step away to take advantage of her brainpower during silence to cultivate her higher-level strategic thinking capacity and to generate, thought-filled original ideas to lead discussions in upcoming briefings. Based on published research findings, I told Betsy that if she strengthened her integrated thinking, I expected the gains would likely spill over to enhance her memory as well. I recommended that we monitor whether or not she rewired her synthesized thinking capacity to a higher performance level and also check for gains in memory function at the same time. Additionally, I found that she had not made time for active exercise in the past few years; thus, I strongly encouraged her to exercise aerobically at least three times per week for approximately one hour. My team and I have found significant improvements in memory function and increased brain volume in brain memory areas in Thinkers who exercise regularly.

Thinkers' Intellectual Capital

As a Thinker, you seek to be the first to know what to do to increase your brainpower. What should you avoid to make sure you are not spending

> Keystone cognitive capacities can be retained and even strengthened with age.

169

unnecessary effort on less consequential areas? What is happening to your frontal lobe functions? What can you do to exploit and invest in your greatest asset and natural resource—your brain?

Certain cognitive functions obviously decline with age, but now we're identifying core cognitive assets that can be retained, regained after losses, and even strengthened.

Thinkers want to know:

- How much intellectual capital have you built up?
- What are the best brain investments—which areas are the most profitable?
- How can you best hedge your bets to make sure your intellectual savings represent a balanced brain portfolio to protect against the potential doom and gloom losses versus preventable decline?
- What mental activities are time wasters instead of brain savers?

Increasing Intellectual Capital in Thinkers

Thinkers, do not despair. New findings reveal that you have immense potential to be as sharp as or even sharper than you were decades earlier on dynamically complex cognitive processes. What age do you think most CEOs of major corporations are? **If mental capacity peaked in early adulthood, then CEOs predictably should be young adults—right?**

The peak age of CEOs for Fortune 500 companies are in the Thinker age group. Conversely, there are nearly zero CEOs forty and under.

The steep downward slope in cognitive losses[16] does not correspond to real-life abilities to reason and deal with crises. The cognitive tests used in the majority of cognitive aging studies do not capture the intellectual capital or the potential required to be successful in the complexity of responsibilities that increase with age. My team and others are revealing that **age alone,**

if one remains healthy, explains only a very small proportion of what is changing cognitively.

I am not surprised that in accounting for cognitive ability, Timothy Salthouse, a renowned expert on cognitive aging at the Department of Psychology, University of Virginia, proposes that age contributes only 20 percent at most to cognitive losses. Supporting a newly arising view of cognitive growth with age, I found that Thinkers rate their peak performance as being right now—not in the past—on the complex cognitive processes necessary to tackle everyday responsibilities.

Check out your perception of your peak performance on key issues relevant to high-level cognitive functionality. Fill out the following questionnaire we developed in partnership with the MetLife Mature Market Institute to assess how people view their brain status.

Check the time when you were/are/will be at peak performance in the following areas:

	In the past	Now	In the future
A. Taking time to think about possible good and bad outcomes of situations			
B. Using information from different areas to come up with new ways to solve problems			
C. Working toward a common goal despite opposing viewpoints			
D. Actively acquiring knowledge to make complex decisions			
E. Orchestrating the steps required to carry out a vision			
F. Feeling confident in your decision making			

Now compare your responses to a group of recently surveyed Thinkers (ages forty-six to sixty-five) who responded to an online survey sponsored by MetLife Mature Market Institute,[17] conducted in 2011—the first year the boomers were turning sixty-five.

Overall (All Boomers)

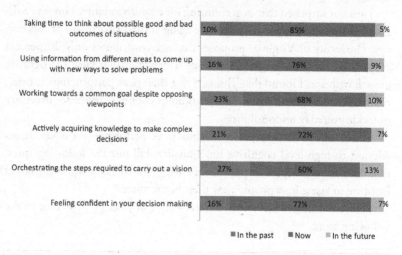

	In the past	Now	In the future
Taking time to think about possible good and bad outcomes of situations	10%	85%	5%
Using information from different areas to come up with new ways to solve problems	16%	76%	9%
Working towards a common goal despite opposing viewpoints	23%	68%	10%
Actively acquiring knowledge to make complex decisions	21%	72%	7%
Orchestrating the steps required to carry out a vision	27%	60%	13%
Feeling confident in your decision making	16%	77%	7%

As you can see from the graph above, a majority of your group perceive their dynamic fluid thinking capacity to be optimal now—or expect it to improve in future years. Few believe your best brain years to be behind you in younger days. The items were selected to elicit personal reflections about how Thinkers view their peak performance on keystone frontal lobe functions of reasoning, learning, planning, adapting, and confidence in decision making. You can see an obvious omission about memory. In earlier studies at the Center for BrainHealth in more than six hundred adults, Thinkers always responded that their memories were better in the past. **Memory is important, but how a person strategically manipulates information is more vital than how much one remembers.** Would you rather be able to quickly remember an obscure date or know how to talk to your parents' doctor to help them receive the proper medical care?

As a Thinker, you are a bit conflicted. When asked what age your brain was the sharpest, you typically say at least ten to twenty years ago, suggesting your best brain days are behind you. On the questionnaire above, many of you said now. And then you go on to characterize your younger decision-making days in these ways:

- Rarely taking the time to weigh the pros and cons of actions when younger
- Not thinking much about how things went to consider new solutions
- Not thinking through where others might be coming from
- Not really thinking about mistakes except to feel bad—not how one could learn from them

Only a very small portion of your group felt your peak performance to be in the past. When I compared the younger boomers/Thinkers (ages forty-seven to fifty-three years) to the older boomers/Thinkers (sixty to sixty-five years), there was a significant difference in the query about "orchestrating the steps required to carry out a vision." Approximately 40 percent of the older boomers/Thinkers felt their peak performance on this dynamic ability of envisioning and completing a goal to be in the past, when they were younger. I can see why that might be true—with increasing age, we may become less inclined to attend to the tedious aspects required to make the big things happen. Perhaps we get used to delegating and lose confidence in making sure all the necessary steps are completed, for good or bad.

In sum, the responses from more than a thousand boomers/Thinkers argue against the view that the majority of your generation feels you fall short in dynamic reasoning and problem-solving aspects related to everyday life. You appear confident in your cognitive abilities to:

- deal with novelty.
- effectively accumulate new knowledge that requires more than manipulating old learnings.
- flexibly weigh consequences from either potentially positive and negative outcomes.
- make competent decisions.

Despite these relatively high ratings for adequate brainpower, it is important that as a Thinker you do not slough off and become satisfied with the status quo of your brain function. Like Jim Collins, a leading American business consultant, author, and lecturer who wrote the book *Good to Great*, says, "Good is the enemy of great" as applied to business practices where companies fail to transition to great as they become complacent with status quo of good enough.[18] **Nowhere is the saying "Good is the enemy of great" more applicable than in brain functionality.** The goal is to push beyond adequate brain capacity, continuing to recognize and act on the need to strengthen and increase your intellectual capital regularly.

Strength Assessment in Intellectual Capital

For years you have maintained annual physician visits, and according to a 2008 report from the Institute for the Future, the baby boomer generation holds the status of the healthiest generation in American history.[19] The word "aerobics" was coined during the Thinkers' early pivotal years. This health obsession has focused mostly on physical health because we have not been long aware that much, if anything, could be done to increase brain health and intellectual capital.

> A Thinker's idea of fitness stops at the neck.

As a Thinker, you are always the first to ask questions and say you want to know everything about what you should be doing for your brain's health. On the flip side of that, you are also slow to follow through on getting new information, mainly due to the *fear* that resides in your mind of what memory concerns could mean. Plus, you hold on to the belief that what you don't know won't hurt you. You still widely believe your intellect is largely fixed and immutable, but that is a false concept that has been held far too long to the detriment of those who have been told they are average at best.

Instead of being frozen by fear, you should start investing daily in your brain's health. The news is comforting and compelling. Based on Brain-Health Physical results, we find Thinkers' cognitive performances to be holding up well on the three core cognitive areas of:

- Strategic attention
- Integrated reasoning
- Innovation

On the domain of strategic attention, the Thinkers' performance is superior to the Seekers (younger adults) and the Knowers (older adults). They spontaneously adopted the strategy to block out information to make their learning efficiency higher. But all three groups learned to efficiently apply strategies to improve learning with repetition.

Let me also interject that not all Thinkers are equally at the top of their brain game. Some brains hold up better than others. Group data obscures and both under- and overestimates performance by individuals. Approximately 30 percent of the Thinkers had vulnerabilities on strategic attention. Similar group profiles of cognitive stability were also identified for integrated reasoning and innovation in Thinkers. That is, Thinkers seem to maintain the ability to synthesize meaning and to create a large number of novel interpretations. For both domains, 30 percent had lower performance, but individuals who exhibited lowered capacities were not all the same across all three domains. As expected, memory performances were lower than core frontal lobe abilities. Identifying which areas can and should be boosted with investment capital will inform brain health practices and training development.

Brad is a perfect example of a talented Thinker who may need to rebalance his brain health portfolio. Brad is a fifty-five-year-old entrepreneur who received his MBA from Columbia and has launched and mentored more than twenty new ventures and businesses. He commented that his concentration powers had changed in that he could not concentrate as long as he used to, but he felt his depth of reasoning was better than ever. He judged that he was able to extract the necessary business details to determine whether he felt different ventures were viable businesses. Once he had carefully thought out the bigger strategies, he was able to adeptly conceptualize the steps to carry out the vision.

> Are your cognitive investments in frontal lobe assets as strong as they need to be?

On the BrainHealth Physical, he exhibited some interesting patterns on the three core frontal lobe functions. On strategic attention, he performed almost at the highest level possible on the first two trials. He selected predominantly the most important items and blocked out the irrelevant data. But on the third trial, his performance completely broke down and he was no longer strategic. He was equally selecting important and irrelevant items to recall. He went from being a Quick Study–Strong Strategic Attention pattern responder to a Strategy-less Inefficient Strategic Attention responder (individuals who try to remember everything without applying a strategy, failing to focus particular information while ignoring other less relevant information). It is unusual to see someone's performance slip so abruptly, but Brad obviously had overloaded his working memory. As he himself admitted, his ability to concentrate had shortened over the years, but when it was good, it was very good. To combat this deficiency, it was recommended that Brad take frequent breaks when engaging in strategic thinking activities to maintain high levels of performance.

On integrated reasoning, he relied more on the literal input than on constructing novel synthesized ideas from his wealth of expertise and prior knowledge. This frontal lobe asset was vulnerable and likely needed fine-tuning to make sure no more slippage occurred. In contrast, Brad was an impressive performer on innovation. He exhibited flexibility of thinking, offering multiple solutions and rich interpretations. Brad can continue to strengthen his brain investment by being tuned in to when his filter was being breached and stepping away to let his brain rest.

Balancing the Brainpower Portfolio

One of **the greatest assets of your Thinker generation is your deep repository of learned information and experiences that accrue extensively each year if you stay mentally engaged.** This yearly brain gain builds and protects your intellectual assets.

Hedging Your Bets

Cognitive neuroscientists are on the cusp of more fully recognizing how Thinkers can increase their mental astuteness. These discoveries will help identify the steps Thinkers can take to make the best investments that will pay off in terms of increased cognitive brain fitness.

Look at Bill Gates, Condoleezza Rice, and Bill and Hillary Clinton—all of these Thinkers are still climbing to reach the peak of intellectual power. Indeed, as a group, your brainpower as a Thinker can continue to be cultivated and nourished to maintain healthy cognitive function for years to come.

Thinkers, take notice: You can nurture and improve your mental productivity by strengthening frontal lobe power—powers that were

difficult, even next to impossible, to master at younger ages. **Frontal lobe functions are a promising path to increasing intellectual capital.**

Human frontal lobe functions may be modified in both good and bad ways as you age. The trick is that these networks must remain exercised and challenged to retain high levels of competence. The more you engage these rich information associations, the more likely you are to retain and increase higher brainpower and strengthen the complex brain network. The saying "A brain that rests will rust" applies to frontal lobe functions.

> Thinkers: Change the course of your own brain health, build cognitive reserves, regain losses, and even stave off what you may deem inevitable cognitive decline if you practice healthy brain habits regularly—daily.

Increasing Investment in Strategic Attention Capacity

Let's face it: memory becomes more fragile as you age. You cannot learn or remember everything—nor should you. What forms of learning build more resilience and be longer lasting? As a Thinker, you can increase their intellectual capital by continuing to master your strategic attention capacity. With age, adults should become increasingly proficient at knowing what to remember and what to discard. Thinkers should actively strive to strategically gauge what to learn and what to block. Improving performance in this domain will make your brain more efficient at learning and remembering.

Take Yvette, a fifty-seven-year-old top executive of a nonprofit company. She scored high on measures of integrated reasoning and innovation. In terms of integrated reasoning, she demonstrated robust function during her benchmark assessment. She was able to synthesize and apply meanings from new content to broader contexts. And on innovation, she showed very strong brainpower and was able to develop innovative, novel ideas.

But her strategic attention was not up to par with her other frontal lobe functions. She needed to boost her brainpower in strategically gating information. She was frying her brain trying to absorb everything possible as she had been able to accomplish when she was younger. Now the overwhelming amount of information she was trying to absorb was robbing her brainpower. In contrast to Betsy, described earlier in the chapter, Yvette's memory span was above normal. Her problem was that she was trying to take it all in and not triage any information out. She had difficulty blocking irrelevant information. By training Yvette on the three brainpowers of strategic attention (see chapter 4)—the brainpowers of none, one, and two—she was able to strategically attend to critical information and block out unimportant information, an essential skill needed for success in the high-stress environment in which she works. She was surprised to find how energized she was after making this change.

Increasing Investment in Integrated Reasoning

As a Thinker, you often over-obsess about annoying memory glitches. In Betsy's case, her concerns were beyond bothersome, but fortunately they were not impacting her decision making, at least not at the moment. To increase intellectual capital, certain core aspects of memory can be retained and even increased if properly invested. People want to immediately know what part of their memory can get better. Your brain is most efficient at remembering abstracted big ideas and less efficient when it tries to remember lower-level details. These global ideas—deeper, synthesized meanings—are more robustly stored and retrieved.

People value photographic-like memories, which are more precise when we are young, but these exact memories do not correspond to CEO brainpower. That is, **the more you know does not make you a more effective leader.** Thinkers may not solidly remember the specific details of meetings, readings, or speeches, but they should get better and better at remembering the bigger thoughts and directions.

> Thinkers are better at constructing generalized, synthesized meanings than ImMEDIAtes, Finders and Seekers, and Knowers.

One of my Thinker friends, a partner in a successful law firm, recently shared his take on the difference between the young brain and older brain: "I am so glad you clarified what is happening to me and my brain. I was getting so down on my mental capacity. I used to be able to remember every single data point and decision on legal cases—now I cannot remember them to save my life. Our firm is hiring these crackerjack smart young attorneys, and they can take reams of documents home and come back the next day and give me every piece of information I could possibly need. They are remembering circles around me."

Then I asked him, "But can they write a brief to make the case like you?"

He jerked his head back with a knowing look in his eye and replied, "You've got to be kidding! Not even close! They do not even know where to start in making the case arguments. They cannot take the prior cases and abstract the relevant points."

Case closed! Thinkers are able to extract the big ideas and know what details are needed to support the major points. This is not yet true for the younger developing minds. As a Thinker, you will continue to get smarter if you invest in complex thinking.

Remember Betsy, who had horrible memory but strong integrated reasoning ability? Based on my research, I recommended that she work to increase her intellectual capital, not by increasing her weak basic memory, but by strengthening and building her high aptitude in applying knowledge, flexibly synthesizing new learnings, and extending to innovations. As these strengthen, I fully expect her memory to improve. Additionally, I said one of the most effective ways to improve memory is to write down the key things you need to remember in a consistent place.

And then there's Roger, a late-forties middle-level manager. Roger was relatively unconcerned about his cognitive brain function, but he wanted to know if there was some area he might need to improve. He reported a few brain glitches when I first met him, explaining that perhaps they were due to a "constant state of mental overload at work." His days were filled with meeting after meeting and he had a hard time keeping track of all of the information being thrown his way.

Roger gave a solid performance on his brain benchmark assessment in the areas of strategic attention. He was able to block out distractions and focus on important information. But in terms of integrated reasoning, Roger had difficulty going beyond the literal facts to synthesize abstracted meanings. As I encouraged him to take a more global perspective, his ideas became more superficial—a sign of a brain on automatic pilot. He was unable to zoom out or zoom deep and wide (chapter 5). With practice and concerted effort of heavy brain lifting, Roger could change his track. I have not yet seen Roger back for his reassessment to see if he is taking the challenge—perhaps this is not a good sign.

Just like body fitness, you do not have to be in trouble to take steps to increase your brain fitness. The three core frontal lobe domains of strategic attention, integrated reasoning, and innovation require regular practice to stay in top working order.

Increasing Investment in Innovation

Although individuals tend to believe that you either have innovative capacity or not, you learned in chapter 6 that you have great potential to become more innovative every year. Thinkers, however, are most guilty of letting creative thinking fall by the wayside instead of continuing to sharpen this critical skill.

> As a Thinker, boiling your problems down to memory issues may make you miss the real culprits robbing your brain value.

Take Mary, a sixty-two-year-old who travels two to three days every week for work. When I first met her, she described her memory as "okay" but was concerned that deficits were detrimentally affecting her ability to carry out her daily tasks. She was beginning to lose her enthusiasm for a job she once coveted and felt energized by. Upon assessment, she demonstrated robust function in strategic attention and integrated reasoning. In these two domains, Mary's brain was operating as a superstar. In contrast, her innovative thinking was abysmal and stilted. Environmental factors were drowning out the creative thinking that fuels the brain. Overloaded by stress, her brain was fried. With a constant flow of information, increasing responsibilities, nonstop travel, and the drastic time difference she had to manage with projects all over the world, her brain was taxed; she was on overdrive and automatic pilot. Mary struggled to come up with new ideas and ingenious ways to interpret approaches beyond what was already in practice. She has stopped stretching her innovative spirit to change things up, as she was using up all her energy just to survive her strenuous schedule. We will continue to advise her, providing strategies to help her regain her innovative brainpower. The potential could be dormant or it may be temporarily weakened (aka a "stress fracture").

These cases demonstrate the difference in brainpower under varying circumstances. Each individual had the capacity but did not know how to tap the well of the brain to maximize his or her potential.

In a recent randomized study of brain training versus physical training for Thinkers, my team and I found that innovation was the area that experienced the greatest gains in brain training. We also found that innovation improvements added to the confidence the participants felt in their cognitive ability and diminished depressive symptoms even in the absence of clinical depression.

> Increasing innovative thinking will be one of the most promising investments to increase intellectual capital.

Will the Intellectual Reserves Hold Out Through Retirement Age?

The majority of Thinkers live in fear that their bodies will outlive their minds. The stats for onset of dementia are frightening, given that an estimated one of two who live to be eighty years and older are likely to develop some form of dementia. Thinkers have seen their parents struggle with loss of mental function in growing numbers, witnessing firsthand the high economic costs of loss of brainpower. Thinkers have had to step in to make the complex decisions for their parents. In some cases, Thinkers' financial resources are burdened or even depleted due to the costs of elderly parents whose cognitive resources fall short.

The Brainomics of Thinker Brainpower

The brainomics of longevity are an immense concern to individuals and public policy experts. Will there be enough money to support the massive numbers of Thinkers who are reaching retirement age, especially if their brain health does not allow independence and personal decision making?

Thinkers have been satisfied living as fully in the present as possible, taking advantage of all the amazing opportunities before them. The world has truly

181

been your oyster as you achieve educationally, travel internationally, rapidly climb the business ladder of success, reinvent yourselves in terms of job and life skills, and even embrace relocating. These vast prospects of growth and change were rarely attainable or sought after in earlier generations.

Only recently are you beginning to think about your future and its sustainability. Your concerns have focused largely on whether you will be able to retire as young as you had hoped, typically on or before the age of sixty-five. That is, you have been most anxious about whether you have the financial wherewithal to maintain the lifestyle to which you have become accustomed.

Whatever our age, our human cognitive capital is our greatest natural resource if properly mined (chapter 7). Thinkers spend little time pondering whether they have the brainpower to sustain their functional independence and personal decision making. Mainly this void exists because you believe you were born with the level of brainpower or intelligence you would always possess. If you believed it possible to improve, you would be all over it.

> Brain concerns for Thinkers should supersede money matters since the latter can be solved if you pay attention to the former.

Thinkers also experience the personal **brainomics** of the high economic costs of stalled brainpower development in your children. You are often referred to as the sandwich generation, as you are not only having to support aging parents but also your children who are taking more years than ever to graduate from college. With college tuition at all-time highs, there are large costs to educating your children. Today our young adult children are returning home after college in record numbers because their brainpower and a dismal job market are not leading to self-sufficient employment or life sustenance.

Thinkers have always felt mentally competent. Consequently, you have not stopped to realize that your own brainpower may require your immediate and constant attention. You may not be building the necessary reserves for a sustainable brain future. The **brainomics** of Thinkers is rapidly diminishing. That is, Thinkers' own insidious cognitive brain decline may become an even costlier reality than what you have been doling out for your parents and children combined.

Take Bart, a fifty-two-year-old recently widowed dad, working full-time as an attorney and serving as primary caregiver to three children. When I met him, he reported living in "overdrive" and consistently "pushing to the limit."

He said he had difficulty sleeping and only averaged two to four hours a night. To combat consistent fatigue, he downed eight cups of coffee a day! Although he found time to exercise every day and followed a moderately healthy diet, his daily grind took its toll. Lack of sleep combined with personal and professional stress caused emotional problems such as depression, anxiety, and panic attacks.

Before his BrainHealth Physical, Bart reported poor memory for day-to-day information and had difficulty concentrating and organizing his thoughts and words into clear communication. What we found during his assessment was an ability to identify the main ideas of information, but his ability to communicate those ideas was fragmented and lacked sufficient supporting information, making it difficult to understand his meaning.

For Thinkers, now is a vital time to build your brainpower. Doing so will not only improve your brain's function now but will also contribute to your cognitive reserves to stave off cognitive decline. Reread chapter 5 to more fully recognize and embrace your potential and the immense brain health gains from regularly engaging in complex mental activities such as integrated reasoning. You will strengthen and maintain high brain performance; your overall brain will be healthier with promises of increases in brain blood flow, increased communication between brain regions and strengthened synapses.

Good brain health habits to adopt:

1. Take inventory of all that goes on in your life and figure out ways to take control of your brain function. Figure out what makes you inefficient and drains your brainpower and come up with ways to mitigate things that take their toll.
2. Exercise your gatekeeping skills on a constant basis. Each day, prioritize and find ways to delegate or eliminate tasks.
3. Despite your drive to respond to inquiries and communications in a timely manner, it's important to consider that efficiency can be the enemy of excellence. Take your time when processing information and composing responses to emails. Allowing complex decisions to simmer over time leads to better outcomes.
4. Try to focus on one thing at a time, especially when you're

dealing with complex issues. A chaotic environment is counterproductive for remembering detailed information and for the deeper-level processing that is required for creative problem solving and troubleshooting.

5. Take time to think about information and synthesize it into the most important ideas. Make sure what you write is a balance between high-level ideas and relevant detail. Writing down important and big ideas can be helpful when considering the sheer volume of information with which we are exposed, and this is also true for the important detail-level information you receive. Not every detail is important, but the ones that are critical are worth documenting, especially when you have to keep lots of balls in the air.

What are you waiting for? You alone have considerable control over the destiny of your brain's health. If you are a Thinker, you will be motivated to ramp up your brainpower today.

Know Brainers

1. Thinkers will reap the greatest investment gains when you invest in your frontal lobe assets more than your memory capacity.
2. Thinkers are losing capacity to quickly process new information and to store and retrieve data.
3. Thinkers have increased potential to become effective cullers of unimportant and irrelevant information by recognizing the most salient concepts.
4. Thinkers can avert the brain drain of memory decline by expanding your ability to synthesize bigger ideas from massive input.
5. Innovation should be stronger in the Thinkers' generation than younger generations if this capacity is continually exercised.
6. Thinkers represent the largest age group of Fortune 500 CEOs.
7. The Thinkers' idea of fitness should focus on brain fitness as much as or more than physical fitness.

CHAPTER 10

THE KNOWERS, 66–100+ YEARS OF AGE

If you are older than sixty-five years of age, you are part of the Knower generation, otherwise known as traditionalists. I labeled your group Knowers because you have the greatest breadth and depth of knowledge and experience. You are able to discern what to quickly know and what to forget or, even better, never to encode. You are more than wise, you have the capacity to take advantage of well-practiced habits of strategic thinking, weighed reasoning, and immense creativity to expand your brainpower and to mentor others. As a Knower, you frame and remember life events in a more positive perspective than when you were younger. The span of Knowers is growing in numbers as life expectancy is increasing.

How will your brain perform at age sixty-five? At age seventy-five? At age eighty-five? At age ninety-five?

What does retirement mean for your brain?

What cognitive areas are requisite for independent decision making and should be strengthened by training?

What mental activities should you practice to maintain, improve brain performance, and even stave off dementia?

How do you capitalize on your intellectual capital from now until the end of your life?

In what areas is your brain capacity outperforming a younger brain?

Ruth continues to lead an active life, both personally and professionally. Despite a number of brain setbacks—chemotherapy and numerous surgeries where she was placed under general anesthesia—she has built the necessary cognitive reserves to continue to innovate effectively.

Ruth demonstrated her robust cognitive capabilities during her brain health fitness assessment. She was able to adopt a strategic plan for many of the tasks to complete them with ease. On the strategic attention measures, she showed a pattern consistent with having **strong strategic attention** as a person who was able to learn over time and to employ frontal lobe strategies to improve her selecting and blocking skills with practice. She performed well on the BrainHealth Physical on measures of integrated reasoning and innovation, showing an impressive depth of processing complex messages. What may surprise you is that Ruth is nearly ninety years old!

When most would consider their best brain years behind them, Ruth exemplifies just the opposite. She is the perfect example that the brain can improve and dynamically perform no matter numeric age. She considers her brain to be in its prime, despite physical frailty.

> Estimates show that Knowers are the fastest growing population worldwide. By the year 2050, nearly one in every six persons is projected to be sixty-five years of age or older.

As people age, the inevitable happens. There is a loss in vitality, dimming of eyesight, fading of hearing, thinning of hair, and increase in wrinkles—not to mention mental sharpness declines in:

- Speed of thinking
- Ability to efficiently utilize new understandings
- Memory
- Quickness in disambiguating

However, it is not all bad news.

In his book *Lastingness: The Art of Old Age,* Nicholas Delbanco, one of America's most revered writers and thinkers, describes the work of great artists and change makers who exhibited remarkable and lasting intellectual talent into late life.[1] Examples are rich. Renoir, despite being severely crippled with arthritis from midlife, painted the very day of his death at the age of seventy-eight. Einstein discovered the theory of relativity in his twenties but did not know what it meant until his seventies. You may remember Mike Mansfield, the longest-serving majority leader of the United States Senate, who was politically active in various capacities until his nineties. Right now these individuals tend to be exceptions rather than the rule.

> As a Knower, you can maintain and even increase your creative capital with continued mental stimulation if you keep your brain fit and are fortunate enough to avoid Alzheimer's.

The idea that retirement is not the golden glory days of daily joy and meaningfulness is gaining traction by some of the world's richest people who are refusing to retire. In a recent global survey of two thousand high-net worth individuals by Ledbury Research, more than 60 percent are not quitting their professions.[2] The good news is that retirement is not just about economic productivity, but also about how individuals can contribute in meaningful ways to society. Daniel Egan, head of behavioral finance for Barclays Wealth Americas, keenly observed that many people make their wealth doing something they love. So why give it up? He calls them "never-tirees." Link that idea with the fact that individuals who work the hardest, are successful in their careers, and love what they do also live the longest, as discovered by Howard S. Friedman, a professor at the University of California, Riverside, and one of the authors of *The Longevity Project*.[3]

Whereas brain scientists disagree about aspects of cognitive function that can be preserved or vulnerable to decline, most all agree that knowledge can be maintained and potentially increased with age. That possibility alone is exceedingly exciting. **What is even more provocative is that older adults are more proficient at picking and choosing what knowledge to store and what to disregard** as compared to younger adults who store more needless stuff—only later to discard. That is, as a Knower, you are selective about what you add to your storage bin, restricting the clutter in your brain's attic.

Despite the capacity to maintain knowledge, as a Knower, you do experience more difficulty recalling particular knowledge at the instant you want it. Nonetheless, the surprising realization is that the memory has not disappeared with advanced aging; it just takes you longer to call it up. The sought-after item or name is usually found, just not timely enough for that usage. Fascinatingly, you remember what you forgot, so it's really not gone—it's just hiding.

Not only does the capacity to hold on to and expand experience and knowledge remain stable with advancing age, the memory for the positive side of events increases with age as well. That is, as you age, you often fail to even encode the negative aspect of events. Against the stereotype of getting more and more negative with age, we, in fact, tend to pay less attention to the negative side of things and are much more likely to remember the good of a situation or context. Cognitive studies show that older adults (at least those not suffering from progressive brain disease) are less likely to dwell on information that has a negative valence—instead showing a much higher preference for positive-valenced information. Moreover, older adults are less likely to display destructive social behaviors such as shouting or name calling[4] in tough emotional exchanges. Negative moody periods are shorter lived in older adults than in young adults. If those are not enough positive trends for you as a Knower, add one more: older adults reconstruct earlier life events in a more positive light than what actually happened.

> Our memory becomes more positive with increasing age.

So when would different age groups say they would be the happiest? This perception of happiness across the age span is exactly what studies by both Laura Carstensen, director of the Stanford Center on Longevity and a professor of psychology, and Peter Ubel, a professor of medicine and psychology at the University of Michigan, tested.[5] They asked a group of Finders (thirty-year-olds) and a group of Knowers (seventy-year-olds) this question. To no one's surprise, both groups solidly picked the thirty-year-olds to be happier. The twist came when they asked both groups to rate their own happiness. The Knowers rated themselves happier by far.

Think about these brain states—*enjoyment, happiness, sadness, worry,* and *stress.* Enjoyment and happiness peak in Knowers. Sadness, worry, and stress are the lowest in Knowers. Who knew that with aging comes increased happiness? Who would have suspected this? The added benefits of Knowers being on the higher end of the happy scale are that happiness has two additional gains: (1) happier people are healthier and (2) happier people are more productive.

Of course, age alone does not explain it all. Individual happiness varies. Consider these questions:

- Do unhappy people die sooner?
- Do older people have more money and therefore worry less?
- Do unsettling teens who have left the house help lighten the Knowers' moods, emotions, and daily burdens?

None of these factors account for the major differences in happiness between groups. Does one give up striving to be something they are not likely to become—skinnier, younger, richer, and happier? Perhaps older people are more relaxed with who they are. As stated above, as a Knower, you tend to have fewer blowups, but even more interesting is that you devise better and more solutions to conflicts. Knowers can definitely be the **more innovative thinkers** in conflict resolution.

> The grayer the world gets, the happier it becomes.

Brainomics of Knowers

Nowhere is the issue of the high costs of brain drain more relevant than in the Knower generation. The truth is, aging is costly. The majority of health-care costs are expended during the last few months to year of life. The longer we live, the more likely we are to suffer cognitive, physical, and/or financial hardships. No matter how positive I paint the potential, there is a reality to aging that is costly.

Alzheimer's disease alone is predicted to double every five-year epoch beginning at age sixty-five. Though we are all going to die, the key to health is to stay as mentally and physically fit as possible and to be prepared for the time when we aren't.

As a Knower, you can expect to live for decades enjoying relatively good physical health—and stronger physical health than any generation before. **Your major concern is of cognitive decline, where your mind does not outlast your body.** Many health-care professionals hold the view that the functional capacity of the brain to engage in sound decision making diminishes relentlessly with advancing age. Supporting this view, some scientific research has shown that decision-making abilities peak in the early fifties—years before retirement, according to David Laibson, an economist and professor at Harvard University.[6] This diminishing decision-making capacity would not be good news for you as a Knower if you view it as an unmodifiable outcome of a long life. Instead, it should motivate you to do as much as possible to improve your odds of reversing these trends.

Robert Wilson, a neuropsychologist at Rush University in Chicago, and his colleagues reported that seniors who were more actively engaged in mentally stimulating activities such as reading newspapers, books, and magazines, playing challenging games like chess, or visiting museums were more likely to retain their intellectual investment.[7] Knowers need to upend the widespread aging bias by taking immediate actions to make a concerted effort to reverse and counteract unnecessary cognitive decline. For you to prosper and flourish as a Knower in our rapidly aging and changing world, you must exploit your greatest assets—your intellectual capital and brain health.

Your brain, as a Knower, retains immense capacity to be strengthened by your efforts. Now is the time to take advantage of your brain's inherent plasticity (chapter 1). Don't let your potential go to waste for a single day. You can lead your cohort of friends to implement the necessary steps to maximize your higher brain performance now. Ignoring this is neither a workable nor a sound long-term solution. In fact, a number of corporations say that many of their Thinkers, i.e., boomers, and Knower-age employees have put their minds on automatic pilot and no longer contribute to corporate strategic thinking. Older Thinkers turned Knowers seem to be viewed (and even perceive themselves) as having little to contribute when it comes to novel and innovative thinking. This frame of mind is off—way off. Time is of essence for Knowers to turn the positive index up to focus on their intellectual potential.

> Age itself is not the major cause of intellectual loss; it is more your failure to remain mentally active.

One of my goals is to raise awareness of the brain's potential with advancing years. **As a thriving society, we must change the negative framing of brain aging and instead harness the full frontal potential of our brain's capacity throughout life (where more wrinkles on the brain, by the way, are** a good thing since brain wrinkles indicate a larger cortex—gray matter!) and more fully strive to achieve the brain potential that is yet to come.

What Does Retirement Mean for Your Brain?

In the new millennium, four generations—Finders, Seekers, Thinkers, and Knowers—are working side by side in the workplace for the first time in our nation's history. Although about 95 percent of Knowers are retired, many are not retiring as young as earlier generations did. Instead, Knowers are seeking to continue to work, often with reduced work hours, according to Lynne Lancaster and David Stillman, authors of *When Generations Collide*.[8] More Knowers want to work longer; the limitation is the lack of jobs in tough economic times and some have not kept their skills relevant to the changing workforce demands. **Knowers who do continue to work tend to enjoy their job and are valued by employers because they are hard workers and extremely loyal,** according to Sally Kane, an attorney and writer of hundreds of career-related articles.[9] Many employees are slowly changing attitudes and policies against forced retirement and instead are hiring and keeping older workers. Nonetheless, some Knowers are certainly working in uninspiring jobs only to pay the bills.

For the most part, as a Knower you are continually pondering when you will retire or should retire if you haven't already done so. "Retirement" is an interesting word—particularly when you think closely at what it might mean for brain health. Some definitions of the word are the "withdrawal from service, office, or business; the act of going away, going into seclusion."

When Knowers begin to think of retirement, they all too often put their brains on retirement mode. Each day is a Saturday, where they rarely tackle tough, novel situations and often are not challenged to offer advice on complex issues and problems in new ways, instead staying quietly on course. While a month of Saturdays can sound like a dream—especially when a fast-paced life has run out of steam—Knowers are now living as retired for

> Retirement is associated with concepts like leaving, quitting, abandoning, exiting, separating, taking off, bowing out, escaping.

longer periods than ever before, and many have cautioned that it's not good for vital brain health.

A 2010 study published in the *Journal of Economic Perspectives* showed that "data from the United States, England and eleven other European countries suggest that the earlier people retire, the more quickly their memories decline."[10] A RAND Center for the Study of Aging and the University of Michigan published a study showing that cognitive performance levels drop earlier in countries that have younger retirement ages.[11] Why is this the case? Retirement often takes you away from an engaging social environment, and social interaction is necessary to increase cognitive reserves. Second, once individuals retire, they are often less motivated to participate in mentally challenging and complex problem finding and solving dilemmas.

In fact, when we look at graphs and the research on cognitive losses—some noticeable declines occur right around the time of retirement. This is when Knowers are beginning to focus on having fun and enjoying the things they couldn't take part in while working. But what if you do not have the mind capacity to plan and orchestrate the things that you want to do for the remainder of your years?

> The retirement age of sixty-five was set when the average life span was sixty-three.

Discoveries now show that your brain retains immense capacity to be modified and strengthened into late life. Unfortunately, habits that build healthier brain function may not be fully realized and adopted, especially with the lack of regularly scheduled work or community service demands that have kept the brain engaged mentally and socially. However, this word of caution does not mean that you have to be working in the traditional sense to avoid mental decline. A brain-healthy lifestyle requires constant cognitive challenge and upkeep to maintain high-level function, but certainly this cognitive challenge can take place with reduced work hours or community service or mentoring opportunities after retirement.

Your mind can be stretched in leisure- as well as work-related activities. These two should not be viewed as mutually exclusive. When you retire from service or business, whether as a Knower or Thinker, you can do much to keep your brain active. It is not only imperative but will add life to your brain and excitement to your life.

Knower BrainHealth Fitness

The brain typically is at its maximum weight around age twenty. For many of us, we wish our body's weight maxed out at twentysomething, instead of the gradual increase of two pounds or more every year. For the brain, more or less weight does not necessarily relate to higher or lower levels of cognitive reasoning or decision-making skills. Over our lifetimes, the brain is constantly being hit with insults or changes that can cause the loss of neurons. The brain circuitry in Knowers, just as with other generations, is continually changing. The brain never stays the same. Some scientists argue that aging causes the atrophy of neurons; others go further to implicate the actual loss of neurons may be our own doing.

Not all the hits to the brain are widely understood. Some of the culprits include hormonal influences, chemotherapy, immune system dysfunction, or general anesthesia, to mention a few.[12–13] Think about Ruth—who was treated for breast cancer with chemotherapy and experienced the foggy aftermath of general anesthesia lasting more than a year post-surgery. She continues to challenge her brain to take on new problems to solve and complex information to learn. Her high-level thinking capacity and independent decision making is decidedly robust and impressive to all who know her.

> As a Knower, you may be recruiting your brain networks in different ways than you did when you were younger.

Despite widespread belief that Knowers are at a stage of insidious brain decline, brains of individuals at this life stage do not manifest widespread loss of neurons as compared to that observed in Alzheimer's disease, brain injury, or stroke.

Brain science dictates that all of our complex, goal-oriented behavior is dependent on a healthy brain and how well its different regions talk to one another—especially the frontal lobe networks. **What cognitive skills the Knowers lose in speed and quantity of learning capacity, they make**

> When thinking power depends on previously learned knowledge, as a Knower, you can excel if you keep your brain fit.

up with rich knowledge, experience, and wisdom. Indeed, Knowers potentially could supersede the Thinkers and Finders in terms of frontal lobe brainpower related to deeper level strategic thinking. The reason that this is not what is currently unfolding is that you **as a Knower may be failing to make the effort to capitalize on your vast brain potential.**

Not Warren Bennis, one of the nation's leading business advisors. Currently in his late eighties, he continues to stretch his intellectual capital. He is an active distinguished professor of management at the University of Southern California and has recently authored a book on leadership, *Still Surprised: A Memoir of a Life in Leadership.*[14] He has published vast pearls of wisdom that say you can challenge your intellectual capital by stretching your mind to interpret or counter. Try these examples:

- Leaders must encourage their organizations to dance to forms of music yet to be heard.
- People who cannot invent and reinvent themselves must be content with borrowed postures, secondhand ideas, fitting in instead of standing out.
- Becoming a leader is synonymous with becoming yourself. It is precisely that simple, and it is also that difficult.
- Taking charge of your own learning is a part of taking charge of your life, which is the sine qua non in becoming an integrated person.

Capitalizing on Knower Brainpower

Rapidly expanding evidence heralds the potential of the remarkable brain plasticity of your brain as a Knower to counteract and prevent the cognitive consequences of brain aging. It will require consistent practice and challenges in deeper thinking. You have immense potential to continue to neuroengineer your brains through new learning and by how you use your brain daily.

Strategic Attention
Knowers typically have the deepest storage of knowledge and they are ahead of the Thinkers in knowing what to ignore at the earliest trial—what is best

not to even learn as well as what to learn. In other words, Knowers know what should be tossed out with the trash and not stored in the brain's attic at all—more so than do Immediates, Finders, and Seekers. As a Knower, with practice you can actually increase your performance as superior selectors and inhibitors. One caveat consistent with extant evidence is that your memory span is the lowest as compared to younger generations. But as I have said before: for intellectual capital to grow, it is not how much you know but how you strategically use what you know. That is where your Knower brainpower can excel.

Integrated Reasoning

Steven Spielberg, the acclaimed director of Academy Award–winning movies, has just turned into a Knower. He is busier than ever making new films, TV series, and being with his family. His products represent a perfectly challenging and fun brain-training activity, as they are always thought provoking and his talents contribute a great deal to brainpower by the nature of movies he directs. He says:

> The magic of movies is that everybody sees them differently. I am always so excited when someone tells me what a movie means to them.

That is integrated reasoning at its core. How many different ways can you synthesize meaning off the screen to apply to real life? Try it—for movies such as *Schindler's List* or *War Horse*. This is one of the three-core frontal lobe processes that Knowers get better and better at.

It is even more meaningful to me that Steven Spielberg collects Norman Rockwell paintings. I have used Rockwell paintings for the past thirty years as rich stimuli in my research because of the deep meaning that each painting portrays.[15] The lessons depicted are ageless, and my team and I have utilized many of these illustrations to examine brain activation when a person is processing the abstract meaning versus the isolated detail. Guess what? Older people show preserved patterns of brain activation when processing synthesized meanings.

Knowers in their eighties and nineties show remarkable preservation in integrated reasoning. We have also shown longitudinally that this ability stays remarkably robust—even in the midst of declines in detail memory that grow larger with age. My research was the first to reveal that cognitively healthy adults eighty years and older demonstrate a remarkable adaptive brainpower to derive a central or deeper meaning in the form of an abstracted interpretation that is maintained in memory over long delay periods.[16–17] This pivotal brain capacity has been shown over and over again to be stable, if not enhanced, in Knowers when they stay mentally active.

Our minds, at any age, but particularly as Knowers, decline when you think like robots—information in and information out without reprocessing and reconciling the new input with what is already known. As a Knower, it is vital for you to continue to create new meanings from contexts or readings. If not, your mind will become almost frozen or lose ground.

> As a Knower, embrace your wisdom and seek to be a master of one or two things rather than a jack-of-all-trades.

Knowers, you will find that you can and do think deeper about areas and contexts in which you are an expert. You make wiser choices about how you spend your mental energies rather than shifting willy-nilly to new areas. The latter course of action, where one learns a little bit here and there, builds fragile and short-lived brain connections. It is your disciplined thinking as a Knower that strengthens your brain capital to prevail over the culprits that could diminish your brainpower in pivotal frontal lobe areas.

Be inspired as a Knower because you can maintain and increase your capacity to engage in integrated reasoning and push yourself to never be satisfied with the status quo. This desire to always be creating something new is a boost to brain health.

Innovation

One viewpoint that needs to be retired is that younger brains are more likely to be innovators.

Take Larry, who at seventy-two started a new company—his fifth, to be exact. Moreover, he launched a major foundation to help advise, mentor, and fund promising new entrepreneurs. Think of the brainpower that will be stimulated in Larry as he evaluates newly emerging high-tech companies. As he is a collaborator, he has of course hired a team to help gather all the information, conduct many of the interviews, and narrow the field.

When he took his first BrainHealth Physical approximately four years ago, he was at the top in strategic attention and integrated reasoning. The one area where he showed preserved but average ability was in innovation. Larry took this news to heart—well, really to brain training. He constantly pursued multiple solutions and ideas every chance he got. Four years later his performance on innovation has almost doubled.

Larry is a Knower and a wildly successful entrepreneur. The age of entrepreneurs has been increasing over the past decade. In fact, according to the Kauffman Foundation, the highest rate of entrepreneurship in American has shifted to Thinkers, extending into early Knowers.[18] Older entrepreneurs have higher success rates than younger high-tech start-ups. What accounts for this age-up shift? Perhaps with age comes:

- Greater accumulated expertise in their fields
- Deeper knowledge of customers' needs
- More years of network supporters, increasing access to financial backers as friends

Knowers have the continued capacity to innovate, envision novel ideas, and make them a reality. A slow brain death comes from ritualistic and mechanistic thinking, no matter the age. Creating novel ideas is the best source of energy for the brain. Creativity, productivity, and innovative thinking thrive much later in life than anyone previously thought.

Cognitive neuroscientists at the Center for BrainHealth are advancing the knowledge of how the brain can continue to be innovative early and late in life. Keeping the mind curious matters immensely at both ends

> Novel thinking can improve, not diminish, with aging.

of the age spectrum, especially at the upper end. I often ask older adults if they could do the work they are doing now thirty, twenty, or even ten years ago. Most know they could not. With age and experience comes richer thinking.

Brain-Training Exercises

Knowers' brains retain the potential for neuroplasticity (capacity for the brain to change) in response to how one engages or fails to engage brain networks during mental tasks—either positively or negatively. Individuals across the life span who have higher levels of engagement in complex cognitive activity show a concomitant reduced rate of hippocampal atrophy in the medial temporal lobe, an area of the brain critical for memory.[19] On the downside, disuse of cognitive skills has been implicated in age-related brain atrophy.

My goal is to inspire Knowers about the many ways they can make their brains smarter—longer. Optimal cognitive training for Knowers entails continual engagement in activities that exert mental challenge that is within the range of cognitive capacity, but is neither too easy nor too difficult. Science offers persuasive and mounting evidence that complex mental activity enhances brain health and reduces risk of dementia. Read back over all the good news about gains from active mental stimulation to enhancing brain health in chapter 5. Guess what? About 50 percent of the research participants were Knowers. Get your mind moving!

> By changing your habitual way of thinking, you will experience your best brain years ahead of you throughout this Knower generation.

Before, the public and health-care professionals did not have a good handle on the best ways to engage the brain. I ask Knowers some of the things they do to keep their mind sharp. They report that they partake in the following:

- Playing bridge
- Learning vocabulary from different languages
- Working on crossword puzzles or sudoku
- Learning to use a computer
- Reading constantly
- Listening to music
- Staying busy
- Trying not to overschedule

- Trying new things
- Looking up topics of interest
- Trying to understand new topics on an elementary level
- Doing crafts

The important idea to recognize is that you will get better and better at whatever you practice, regardless of age. There is nothing a Knower cannot do better with one hundred hours of practice. The limitation to most tasks and activities is that practicing specific tasks makes the person primarily better at the skill practiced, but the brain gains rarely generalize to other skills.

One of the key principles to engage and strengthen frontal brain regions is to make sure the cognitive challenge level is fine-tuned in terms of effort expended. When the challenge exceeds capacity to a large degree, Knowers become overwhelmed, discouraged, and may fail completely and withdraw. When the cognitive challenge is effortless, individuals operate almost on autopilot, which does not appear to be the best approach for maintaining brain health fitness.

Coupled with the fact that each Knower's brain is uniquely designed, prescribing a one-size-fits-all program is challenging. The nature of mental stimulation essential for helping Knowers to become smarter for longer varies from person to person due to the increasing levels of individual differences in baseline cognitive function with advancing age.

My research has shown that for Knowers, the brain responds to the complex mental activity involved in integrated reasoning within a relatively short time.[20–22] By training them to engage their frontal lobe during deeper thinking activities, Knowers report and show improvements in brain and cognitive function. The fascinating feature is that no two Knowers' brains are alike, so perhaps it's not surprising that different patterns of response to brain training would be discovered. Knowers' brains exhibit greater variations from one another than do the brains of of any other generation. That is, as we age, we get more different—not more similar. This increasing diversity is due to the vast differences in experiences that build our brains—no two people have the same life experiences—even identical twins.

It is fascinating that as a Knower you can experience not only stability but also vitality in your brain health throughout your life, if you actively practice the core frontal lobe functions. You will also need to continually seek social and environmental stimulation to maintain cognitive stability with increasing age.

I am actively examining how much brainpower can be attained and regained with brain training. In one study, we considered the cognitive gains of integrated reasoning training in a group of seniors whose mean age was seventy-four. After eight hours of training over a one-month period, the Knowers showed training gains in the integrated reasoning ability—the ability to synthesize meaning—a skill relevant to everyday life and decisions. More important, the findings revealed that the brain-training benefits generalized to untrained measures of other frontal lobe functions, including strategic attention, innovation, and cognitive switching.

Two patterns emerged from this study. First, the Knowers with the lowest baseline ability showed the greatest gain in integrated reasoning. Second, those that were already high performers showed spill-over benefits to other cognitive areas of fluid intelligence. The results are being confirmed in a clinical trial where the participants are randomly placed in either a physical training group, a brain-training group, or a wait-list control group.

The early results show that brain training and physical exercise contribute very different gains to intellectual capital. Again, our brain training showed gains in the three core frontal lobe domains as contrasted with memory gains in the physical exercise group. We are looking at changes that look promising for both training groups, but in distinct brain areas. Just think about how little time and effort was required to produce significant brain gains. The problem is that the brain habits likely need to be maintained to keep the benefits. Once you stop complex thinking habits, your brain is at risk for decline.

As you age, ask yourself if your frontal lobe functions are what they should be and what they optimally could be. As a Knower in your seventies or older, take the brain challenge to guard against the notion that cognitive brain decline is inevitable. The brain does change with normal aging, but the changes are not all bad, and with proper focus you can make your brain even better in pivotal cognitive domains than in its younger days.

A Knower's brain has the potential to continually increase its capacity to get better at formulating an informed, experienced position or opinion because of our rich experiences and knowledge. Knowers can also grow to know what questions to ask to prove or disprove a position. Finally, Knowers have the greatest degree of insight into how best to interpret the answers with the greatest positive gains. That is wisdom. It is a brain thing that matters.

Know Brainers

1. Your brain gets more positive as you get older.
2. Knowers can maintain core frontal lobe functions of strategic attention, integrated reasoning, and innovation given continual challenges.
3. Engaging in complex mental activities will likely be associated with considerable gains in neural health and higher cognitive performance.
4. Knowers who are at the top of their mental game should continue to challenge their thinking to keep from going backward.
5. Retirement from work does not have to be a brain loss, but maintaining brain function in retirement will require a concerted effort to pursue social connectedness and cognitive complexities.
6. Knowers can get better and better at solving conflicts due to positive-bent and broad perspectives.
7. Knowers must maintain active mental lifestyles to extend their brain spans to more closely match their life spans.

SECTION IV

MIND THE GAP IN INJURY AND DISEASE

Most consider only the negative of a brain injury or brain disease, but it is also important to remember that injury or disease does not necessarily mean drastic changes or the end of life as we know it. It is vital to keep the brain active in areas of preserved cognitive function and slow cognitive changes. The brain's incredible ability to grow, change, rewire, and repair itself throughout our lifetime offers hope where little existed before.

CHAPTER 11

REBOUND AND REWIRE YOUR BRAIN AFTER INJURY

What is a brain injury?
How is the brain affected by a brain injury?
Why is a concussion considered to be a brain injury?
Can the brain heal after injury?
What is the time window when the brain can be repaired?
Is a brain injury in a child the same as one in an adult?

Thirty-one-year-old Charlie suffered debilitating brain damage because of a car accident. A husband and father of three, he was left unable to think or talk clearly. His doctors told him that he needed to realistically accept that his employment capabilities were low. Discouraged and disappointed, Charlie worried about how he would provide for his young family.

After little progress over eighteen months, Charlie joined one of my studies. After testing him, I discovered that though his language was significantly impaired, his mental capabilities were remarkably strong. To help him achieve optimum brain recovery, I encouraged him to enroll in college classes to ensure that he was continually cognitively stimulated. To his surprise, Charlie surpassed everyone's expectations. Charlie not only received his diploma but also earned magna cum laude honors.

How can such a complex organ like the brain be repaired after injury?

I am frequently asked this very question when I tell Charlie's story during a lecture or public talk. The repair is not the result of a surgical procedure or a medication. It is not a product of a single effort. The astounding ability of the brain to grow, change, heal, and restore cognitive capacities is due to its remarkable plasticity in response to complex mental challenges such as those exemplified in chapters 4, 5, and 6. Yes, these same strategies work in the presence of a brain injury. Acknowledging and taking advantage of this extraordinary ability after injury will not only boost the personal well-being and financial bottom line of those directly affected by injury, it will also positively contribute to the community and nation as a whole.

> We can harness our brain's inherent plasticity to rewire it after injury.

To understand how the brain can repair and restore after injury, you must first understand what constitutes a brain injury.

What Is a Brain Injury?

Brain injury is the loudest silent epidemic. It is alarmingly the number one cause of disability and death in our country and across most other developed countries. It is a leading cause of disability, affecting the lives and livelihoods of nearly two million people in the United States every year.[1-2] It is referred to as silent because you cannot see a brain injury. For the most part a person looks perfectly normal—they walk, they talk—but inside they feel the difference.

> Brain injuries are known as invisible injuries.

- Children who have suffered brain injuries have said they often feel overwhelmed by information.
- Young adults who had injuries earlier in life say they cannot absorb content as fast as their peer group despite feeling as smart as others.
- Older adults often complain that their thinking is just not the same.

- Retired professional athletes talk about feeling like they're in a fog all the time.
- War veterans reflect how often they feel that their minds fail them, leaving them unable to quickly scan and assess the complex environments in which they operate.

What Happens to the Brain in a Brain Injury?

> No head injury is too severe to despair of, nor too trivial to ignore.
> —Hippocrates

Our Brains: Vaulted but Vulnerable

Our amazing brain controls everything we do—our thinking, decision making, ability to make and maintain friendships, capacity to problem solve and figure out best next steps, and more (see chapter 2). All regions of the brain work in concert, like a world-class orchestra, to produce the simplest and most complex activities with seemingly little exertion. When you think about the brain's daily accomplishments, it is literally mind-boggling.

By design, the human brain inhabits a uniquely protective environment; it is hidden away in a vault. To understand a brain injury, it helps to know a bit about how the brain is encased for safety but also how that design is easily breached, and often violated. The vaultlike protection in which our brain thrives has three layers of protection:

- A tough membrane-like cellophane wrap (the dura mater) covers the brain.
- A closed chamber of fluid (the cerebrospinal fluid) surrounds the brain.
- A one-quarter-inch thick bony surface (the skull) encapsulates the brain.

Unlike most other organs, the brain:

- is not fixed in place.
- floats in fluid inside the skull surrounding it.

• is restrained to a small degree by being attached to a long stem—the spinal cord.

Picture a flower floating in the wind. As the wind blows, the delicate flower rotates, changing direction effortlessly. The brain is similar in that it is free to rotate and move about at the end of a stem. But there is a difference. The brain's movement is constrained by the space it inhabits within the skull.

> **The brain paradox: The three-layer, vaulted, protective design of our brain makes it vulnerable to injury.**

Just imagine the brain safely sloshing within your skull as you partake in the following activities:

• Getting out of bed
• Standing up from the sofa
• Turning your head to look for cars behind you
• Walking down stairs
• Jumping over a water puddle in your path
• Throwing back your head in uproarious laughter, or
• Bouncing on a mountainbike down rugged terrain

With each movement, your brain moves in its fluid encasement.

Next, imagine an egg enclosed in a small jar full of water, moving back and forth, bumping softly against the sides of the jar as you walk along. Sounds pretty safe. Although it's benignly bumping against the walls of the jar, the egg is still intact.

Think what would happen to the egg if you ran at full speed into a wall. The egg would undergo an extreme jolt. You, and the glass jar, would quickly stop moving, but inside, the egg twists and reverberates violently even if the glass jar does not break. What are the chances of the egg coming out unscathed, unbroken without a chip? Slim to none.

Now imagine that egg is your brain.

An Injured Brain

There is horrific jarring of the brain when bodies collide, vehicles crash, heads crush against hard surfaces, or explosive forces propel bodies hard to the ground. Picture a brain when:

- Heading a soccer ball
- Tumbling off a person pyramid at a sporting event
- Being bumped abruptly in your car from behind by some-one driving while talking on cell phone. (It is now estimated that more than 80 percent of collisions happen within three seconds of being distracted, typically by cell phone use.)
- Falling from a standing position without catching oneself. (Falling is the number one cause of brain injuries in older adults.)
- Being tackled by a three hundred and fifty-pound linebacker running at high speed, causing the head to be slammed against hard Astroturf
- Being thrown against hard surfaces in blast-related injuries—from improvised explosive devices (IED), rocket-propelled grenades, or mines

Brain scientists are only beginning to appreciate the full extent to which external forces internally injure the brain, allowing a more precise characterization of brain injuries. When the brain is slammed into a hard, bony skull, it rotates and spins. These rotational forces cause shearing and tearing of many nerve fibers that connect near and far brain regions. This stretching and tearing disrupts and cuts off the ability of different brain regions to communicate effectively. Recollect the far-reaching impact across large communities when electrical wires or telephone wires are cut after a devastating storm. That is comparable to what is going on inside the brain of someone who has suffered a brain injury.

A brain can be injured without either the individual or the people nearby realizing it. Nonetheless, the person may still be able to carry out basic functions. How is that possible? The brain has considerable redundancy built into its complex design, allowing multiple areas to take over new functions when others have been damaged.

For the most part, the wide dispersion of random stretching and tearing across brain connections cannot be detected by commonly used brain scan methodologies and technologies widely available in clinical practice today, especially in milder forms of brain injury. But this insensitivity to concussive brain trauma is likely to change in the near future. Already, new imaging techniques, such as diffusion tensor imaging (DTI), are allowing us to document the major shearing of brain fibers in moderate to severe injuries. In the DTI, scans below, image A shows the corpus callosum fibers that connect both hemispheres in a normal brain.[3] In image B, you can see the severe loss of fibers in an individual who has suffered a severe brain injury. The tiny hemorrhages from the blood vessels may show up on computed tomography (CT) scans taken later as small deposits of iron called hemosiderin (iron from an earlier bleed) appear.

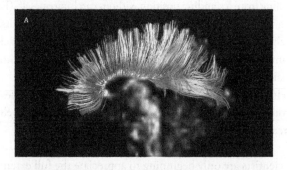

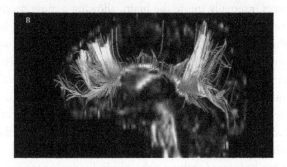

The cascading effects from a brain injury can include some of the following:

  • Brain swelling (edema). Swelling can cause brain herniation
    where the brain is trapped and squeezed against the fixed,
    hard, bony skull. Brain herniation can potentially cut off

blood supply to parts of the brain causing rapid death, even
after seemingly mild injuries
• Increased intracranial pressure
• Seizure activity
• Medication-induced low blood pressure to reduce the high
blood pressure and combat threatening brain swelling
• Hematomas (collection of blood in brain)

These forms of brain disruption can happen in brain injuries of differing
degrees of severity—from the very mild to the most severe.

When the connections deep within the brain are severed or weakened
by tearing, the communication between brain regions is cut off or short-
circuited. As a result, almost all complex tasks that require integration across
multiple brain regions are damaged. Things that were once automatic now
become much more effortful and brain draining.

What are the consequences of a brain injury?

The public has only recently become aware that a concussion *is* a brain
injury, not a benign bruise or bump
on the head. Concussions need to be
taken seriously because potentially
grave consequences may arise as a direct result of such an injury. **Knee and
shoulder injuries receive more medical attention than brain injuries, yet
nothing has more lasting ramifica-
tions than an injury to the brain.** The evidence is clear that persistent
cognitive and behavioral deficits increase exponentially when the brain is
not given time to heal before enduring another concussion.[4] Repair can be
elevated given proper cognitive training even years after the injury.[5]

**True or False? When a concussion occurs, the person is knocked out
momentarily, losing consciousness.**

Most individuals believe this to be true. This perception is what has
guided regulations for removing athletes from play and then returning them
to play for all sports—football, hockey, lacrosse, soccer, basketball, cheerlead-
ing, and even baseball. In reality, rarely does a concussion cause a person to
lose consciousness—whether on the playing field, battlefield, or field of life.

> The frontal lobe is the most
> vulnerable brain region in
> brain injury.

Though the misfortune of a concussion or brain injury is bad, the aftermath is far worse. Throughout my career, I have heard hundreds of gut-wrenching stories of children, teens, adults, and seniors who have experience brain injuries. In each case, **the individual's life as they knew it was dramatically altered in a split second—a change that often has dire ramifications for an entire lifetime.**

> A concussion *is* a brain injury.

Perhaps one of the most **detrimental aspects of a brain injury is that the frontal lobe is the most vulnerable to being damaged,** especially the prefrontal cortex.[6-7] The temporal lobe is the second most commonly injured region. These two regions are the most likely to be injured because the skull areas surrounding these regions have sharp, protruding inner surfaces that act like weapons of destruction as the brain rams against them. Also, the frontal lobe is particularly vulnerable in brain trauma because they have extensively rich long and short connections across and within the deep brain regions. Thus, any stretching and rotating of the brain is likely to disrupt connections to the frontal lobe.

And because of the intricate design of the brain and the command center–like function of the frontal lobe, the rich cognitive strategies a person once had ready for **negotiating and figuring out the complexities of daily life events now become more unpredictable after an injury.**[8] Individuals with mild to severe brain injuries may experience and report symptoms, but health care providers lack the necessary tools or knowledge to detect these complex and debilitating symptoms. **Research reveals that widely used cognitive measures are insensitive to the high-level cognitive deficits in traumatic brain injuries.** In fact, performance on many standardized measures can return to normal or near normal levels of functioning. Individuals are often falsely told the problems should resolve, given time, when they leave the hospital or rehabilitation facility.

My team and other brain scientists are discovering that many may not recover, despite their potential, due largely to:

- premature cessation of training.
- insufficient monitoring.
- ineffective, low-level training protocols.

The traumatic brain injury patient may seem like he or she has returned to normal from the outside—at least when in a familiar, unchallenging environment. **However, after an injury, brain breakdowns erupt unpredictably. When there is a change of expectations or new problems to negotiate, the individual will experience significant cognitive challenges that lead to discouragement and will perplex others.**[9–10] One common outcome is agitation after not being able to overcome the brain inconsistencies.

Despite the return of general normal intellectual capacity in the majority of individuals who suffer a brain trauma, the more lasting consequences of the brain injury will appear as:

- Poor strategic attention to the task at hand in a distracting environment
- Reduced ability to see the big picture to make sound decisions
- Impaired ability to make or initiate a new plan
- Inability to think of solutions beyond the obvious
- Difficulty establishing steps to take from extensive instructions
- Inactivity because one cannot devise multiple solutions to solve a crisis
- Overwhelmed brain when faced with massive input
- Resistant to changing directions
- Inadequate ability to anticipate consequences

If all this sounds like the frontal lobe functions discussed in chapter 2, that's because they are. **Individuals with brain trauma will struggle significantly in dynamically employing frontal lobe functions, as these intricate pathways may be short-circuited and malfunctioning.**

Ryan is a perfect example of a teen who seemed to have recovered from a brain injury. At the age of thirteen, Ryan's life was forever changed when he was hit by a car while riding his bike and was thrown fifteen feet into the air, landing on his head.

Ryan's devastating accident caused dozens of microscopic shearing tears throughout his brain. What may surprise you is that his brain scans did not show any signs of injury. **Ryan and his family were told he would fully recover** from his injuries within months. But a year after his accident, he was still experiencing problems with learning new things. Ryan was having trouble in school and at home. Most research only follows children with traumatic brain injury up to a year after their injuries, but I have been able to document a neurocognitive stall, or a halting or slowing in later stages of cognitive, social, and motor development beyond a year after brain injury. **A pediatric brain injury can be a lifelong process due to the nature of the developing brain.**

The public health issue of how we assess, monitor, and train those with brain injuries will hopefully change rapidly. Research indicates that **many individuals will later show emerging deficits from earlier brain injuries.**[11-12] **I propose that individuals with brain injuries should be monitored on a yearly basis, just like children and adults with a cancer such as leukemia.** Training could be implemented as soon as complex cognitive functions are stalled or later emerging deficits detected in order to ensure that the person "stays in remission" to keep cognitive losses at bay.

The frontal lobe cognitive functions are the most pivotal in terms of supporting our ability to become and remain productive in life. Frontal-lobe-mediated, cognitive-control functions are also the very ones that are most vulnerable to all severity levels of traumatic brain injuries, from mild to moderate to severe.

Repair and Rebound to Get an Edge

After an initial concussion, it's important that the brain heal completely to regain maximum brain performance. Cognitive rehabilitation following a traumatic brain injury traditionally focuses on strengthening specific cognitive skills, such as memory. Doctors and therapists also aim to retrain specific daily functions, such as cooking or driving, through a drill and practice method as well as the use of compensatory tools, such as memory books or planners. Although these training approaches improve targeted skills in acute stages of recovery and are beneficial for short periods, they seldom

> The chances are high that a large proportion of people today will experience a concussion sometime in their lives.

have a significant impact on the quality of life. With many doctors and therapists providing a bleak long-term prognosis, few programs exist that dramatically improve the lives of those with traumatic brain injuries.

As one Navy SEAL I recently worked with stated, "Today if cognitive functioning is increased by 10 percent after an injury, it is considered a success. I argue that a college graduate reading at a third grade level after an injury is not a success; it's an absolute failure. Our men and woman in the military put everything into what they do, sometimes giving their lives for the sacrifice. The organizations responsible for these people spend millions of dollars building, training, preparing them to go into battle. Sadly, no efforts have gone into a focused training regiment for the brain."

It was previously believed that the window for brain recovery was at most one year after injury; my research has shown that the brain can be repaired months and years after injury if the right interventions are applied.[13–15] **Never have I been more optimistic about the potential of the human mind to be repaired**—not only in the short term but, even more impactful, years even decades after suffering brain trauma.

To achieve brain repair at later ages and stages of life, effective treatments and training need to be implemented so individuals can take advantage of restorative brain training now. Unacceptably, the hundreds of thousands who have suffered brain injuries are living with less than their personal best, not rebounding to their maximum, high-performance potential.

The knowledge that the brain can continue to be repaired and strengthened years after injury is not widely appreciated, despite the fact that this information appeared in scientific journals more than a decade ago.

The Power of Plasticity

It has taken so long a time for us to get to this stage for three key reasons:

Technological

Brain imaging technology has improved dramatically over the past ten years, but brain scientists have only recently been able to utilize sensitive brain imaging techniques to measure brain change and brain activation patterns in response to treatments, whether pharmacological or cognitive training. Being able to visibly measure regions of the brain as they start communicating again is extremely encouraging.

Short time windows for brain repair

Widely held tenets of brain repair had previously been limited to only one-year post–brain injury, with the greatest extent of recovery taking place within the first three months. This evidence has provided the guideline to define insurance coverage. At present, most medical coverage runs out within three months after injury, with rare cases extending benefits up to six, maybe twelve months at most. These coverage time intervals have been defined by falsely held brain repair assumptions of limited recovery after one year.[16] The new brain science must be translated and insurance must be revamped and lengthened to achieve higher levels of recovery and long-term productivity.

Training regimens largely ignored rebuilding frontal lobe functions

*Most treatment protocols were focused on specific cognitive processes to achieve basic functions, such as memory or attention. Results of these programs improved the specific skills trained but failed to show significant degrees of transfer to complex skills needed to orchestrate the intricacies of life work and to maintain healthy relationships both within the family unit and beyond. **Until recently, little focus was given to training the dynamic fluid thinking of frontal lobe skills because the mainline thinking of brain repair experts was that training had to start from the bottom to rebuild skills.** Evidence has mounted in present years that basic bottom-up training has not worked. This low-level training focus does little to make sure the individual achieves his or her personal best.*

A focus of my team is to advance brain health and high performance for all individuals who have suffered brain injury. In the near future, we plan to capitalize on new technology platforms to provide virtual diagnostic evaluations and episodic, long-term training wherever the individual is injured or resides—allowing all to be monitored long term and to receive the best training possible by the most talented experts.

Most exciting are the discoveries that significant degrees of brain rewiring and repair can be achieved after training that engages frontal lobe cognitive control processes.[17] Remember Ryan? He participated in training where we taught him how to more effectively assimilate, manage, and utilize information—skills that are crucial for academic success and overall brain function in daily life. We were able to train and monitor his recovery of important cognitive, social, and emotional functioning abilities months after his initial injury.

After training, Ryan showed improvements in several areas, including his ability to interpret and express important ideas from what he was reading, as well as his ability to use critical thinking skills to abstract the deeper-level meanings from complex information. His mother also reported improvements in areas that we did not train specifically, including emotional control, initiation, working memory, planning, and organizational abilities. These are major life improvement gains.

As has happened over and over in my career, the amazing people with whom I work inflame my mind to continuously update my research goals. Scientists at the Center for BrainHealth are searching for ways to:

- increase human cognitive potential.
- enhance brain edge and high performance.
- develop and test new frontal lobe training regimens.
- repair and restore cognitive brain health after injury.
- ensure that those with brain repair achieve their personal best throughout life.

The mechanisms of plasticity can be harnessed to bring about neuronal changes, many of which are beneficial and some of which may not be. The changes are seen at the neurotransmitter level as well as at the most complex level of how different regions of the brain work together to make things happen—including intracellular signaling, cell birth, alterations in dendritic and axonal structures, and more.

The complete answer as to how exactly the brain rewires with use remains to be explored, but we know that it happens and that it takes different routes. Some of the possible ways include these:

- Sometimes the **injured brain region heals;** the function of that region returns to the same brain area.
- At other times, **the areas surrounding the injured area take over** that skill set.

- Another possibility is when **the opposite side of the brain begins to play** an integral role in taking over the functions previously performed by the injured networks.
- It is also plausible that almost new or completely new combinations of brain pathways start to work to support the cognitive processes that have been disrupted.

The brain has immense plasticity to rewire and reorganize. One great example of this is in the research of brain rewiring in persons with deafness.[18] Areas of the brain devoted to hearing were shown to become actively involved in visual processing in deafness. It was revolutionary to discover that a person with severe hearing loss would reorganize his or her brain such that the auditory cortex, no longer actively engaged for hearing purposes, would be called upon to process complex visual spatial patterns—more commonly processed in the visual cortex. Although this explanation is oversimplified, the immense plasticity of the brain is richly illustrated.

Cognitive scientists around the world are actively researching and developing specific approaches to build stronger brain function not only in health, but also in brain injury. Science is investigating ways to substantially advance brain repair through brain training or drugs either used alone or in combination. I expect great gains in the next decade to define ways to measure and achieve cognitive improvements and the underlying brain mechanisms that support these gains.

The rewiring of a brain depends on the degree to which the brain is challenged, just as it does for those with uninjured brains. The power of brain plasticity, especially at stages one year and longer postinjury, depends on the complexity level of the mental challenge and the relevance of the activity to real life. In later years after the injury, the majority of spontaneous brain repair mechanisms have halted or significantly slowed. If a person with a brain injury is trained using predominantly low-level thinking tasks, those are the connections that will be rebuilt. As individuals with brain injury are trained to practice advanced thinking and reasoning, based on our evidence we expect they will rewire frontal lobe networks to support those functions. As the cognitive brain levels are challenged, the brain will rewire networks and make headway in regaining lost or weakened skills.[19]

John Prigg was one of the top high school wrestlers in Texas when he suffered a severe head injury. "John fell underneath the other opponent, hit the side and then back of his head on the wood floor outside the mat. It was an accident. It was devastating," John's father said. Immediately John, his family, and the medical staff caring for him knew his memory had been affected. "It was just a heart-sinking feeling when your son doesn't even know he's a wrestler when he's in a wrestling meet, in his wrestling uniform. That's pretty devastating," John's father told me.

His mother noticed something else, too. "People who did not know my son, they did not know that he was very outgoing—the first one with a practical joke, the first one with a hug, a pat on a back, a little wrestling move. After his accident, he just seemed like a very quiet, shy, withdrawn teenager, and that was not my son."

John underwent extensive therapy to relearn basic activities such as eating and showering. He struggled completing and coherently communicating his thoughts, but he was determined to improve his thinking abilities, to move past his injury and on with his life.

After twelve hours of intensive training five years after his initial injury, John was able to better convey his thoughts and communicate his ideas. As John said, "I feel like I can problem solve and organize my thoughts to achieve a goal." John's scores after training demonstrated his success. His strategic thinking and organizational skills improved by 50 percent. The transformational program provided life skills for improved quality of life, helping John and others like him with traumatic brain injuries think smarter, not harder.

> The time window for brain repair may be limitless except in very severe cases.

Brainomics

The high economic cost of brain loss in injury is exorbitant since we have failed to rebuild stronger brain capacity. The loss is greatest in those with the mildest forms of injury because they:

- are the most likely to return to pre-injury cognitive levels.
- represent the largest proportion of brain injured (approxi-

mately three in four have mild brain injuries). Our research indicates that about 30 to 40 percent of these will go on to have persistent or later-emerging deficits.

• possess a high potential to have a productive life given timely training.

The Brain Injury Association of America reports that "while a price can't be put on the cost of the emotional and physical issues that arise as a result of a brain injury, a price can be put on the financial burden that results from a brain injury. The monetary cost of brain injuries varies significantly—it's estimated that a mild head injury costs $85,000; a moderate injury costs $941,000; and a severe injury costs $3 million. Overall, it is estimated that the cost of traumatic brain injuries in the United States weighs in at $48.3 billion annually."[20]

According to the Centers for Disease Control and Prevention (CDC), acute care and rehabilitation of brain injury patients in the United States costs about $9 billion to $10 billion per year.[21] This does not include the indirect costs to society as well as to families, including the costs associated with lost earnings, work time, and productivity, as well as those linked to providing social services. While costs vary according to the extent of the injury and its specific long-term effects, it is estimated that the cost of caring for a survivor of severe traumatic brain injury is between $600,000 and $1.875 million over a lifetime.

Individuals with concussions and other more severe forms of traumatic brain injury are at risk for not being able to achieve a productive life independently. A survey of traumatic brain injury needs across fourteen states reported that one-third required significant assistance when taken one year post-injury.

It's hard to fathom the widespread degree of stalled brain potential that has occurred from past injuries, not to mention the unacceptable years of of future loss of brain potential if brain training protocols to help victims recover are not converted to everyday practice and brain care. The prior lack of effective long-term treatment offerings was not because the brain could not be repaired. **Rather, the void was a result of the pervasive false perspective that the brain was a rigid organ with limited potential to birth new neurons**—much less new brain connections after injury. The brain was conceived as a fixed black box—instead of an organ with an amazing capacity to continue to change, be modified, and be repaired into late life given proper degrees of cognitive challenges.

> Even small incremental gains in brain performance would make significant cost reductions and, even better, ensure that those with injury continue to be productive in life.

In 2008, Stanley Francis was "pretty banged up" in a motorcycle accident. While wearing a helmet, he was tossed thirty feet into the air, landing face-first. After several hours in the ER, doctors assessed his physical injuries (several broken ribs) and made sure there was no severely acute trauma to the brain. Discharged and thankful to be alive, Stanley went home, and within weeks, back to work.

It was at the office that Stanley first noticed changes in his cognitive function. "I had always been able to keep everything mentally cohesive, but after the accident I struggled with completing thoughts and following through," he said. "I first took note of my struggle with personal interaction during a conference call with a client. I was asked a question that I should have answered diplomatically and thoroughly, but instead I just abruptly brushed it off and changed the subject."

"Immediately after that phone call, one of my colleagues suggested that I look into the long-term effects of traumatic brain injury. His daughter had similar struggles after an injury, so he was knowledgeable about both the effects and treatments," Stanley said.

"After the accident, we focused on getting Stanley's physical ailments healed," his wife, Carol, told me. "It was a full year before any other issues were noticed. Stanley was always gifted in analyzing information, digesting it, and presenting a summary in a very logical manner. Suddenly it seemed that instead of going from point A to point B in a straight line, he would start, then wander around in circles, maybe never arriving at point B at all. Even more, his usual mild-tempered personality was now vacillating between passive and aggressive."

After an initial appointment with a clinical neuropsychologist, Stanley was referred to the Center for BrainHealth, where researchers employed strategies with a goal of teaching participants how to better enhance strategic attention, integration of information, and innovation. The methodology and strategies are designed to improve frontal lobe flexibility and function.

"I was very skeptical at first," Stanley said. "The processes we were learning seemed, to me, too simple to have an effect. But after the second session, they began to work."

In just eight sessions, Stanley began to notice improvements in how he was thinking, his depth of responding, and his problem-solving skills in both his personal and professional lives. Since completing the study, he has made the strategies integral parts of his daily routine. "It's been profound," he said.

Stanley continued, **"I didn't want to be defined by my traumatic brain injury,** and if I had not completed the program, I wouldn't have the strategies I need to manage my daily life."

If you have experienced a brain injury recently or years ago, here are a few tips to help you take advantage of your brain's capacity to rewire:

1. **Keep a balanced level of brain stimulation.** When your brain has been injured, active mental stimulation is required to continue to recover lost cognitive functions and to repair the brain. A word of caution is that the mental challenges should not be too low or too high, otherwise your brain will shut down with boredom or agitation. The tasks need to be ratcheted up a notch constantly to achieve brain rewiring.

2. **Strengthen strategic attention.** When the brain has been injured, some abilities are particularly degraded and compromised. To compensate:
   * Keep background stimulation as low as possible. The brain has to work harder to comprehend and quickly process input while simultaneously actively blocking out extraneous distractions. The brain after injury tires quicker especially when you do not minimize stimuli intruding on your thinking.
   * Avoid trying to do two things at once. This is more difficult after a brain injury, so focus on one task at a time.
   * Identify your top two tasks; get help if needed. The brain gets quickly overwhelmed when given a long to-do list.

3. **Practice integrated reasoning.** After a brain injury, the brain

quickly shuts down when it has too much detailed information. Practice restating or writing down your big ideas. This provides experience in synthesizing meaning continually. This practice will increase levels of brain repair and mental productivity tremendously. Integrated reasoning will also likely transfer to higher levels of functionality in everyday life.

4. **Never give up.** Your brain can continue to rewire for the rest of your life. Keep looking for new ways to challenge your mind to repair and to reach higher levels of recovery.

5. **Expect new breakthroughs each year in brain repair.** Keep researching to stay in touch with new scientific discoveries that may promote brain rewiring. **Reach out to experts who can offer advice as to the next steps** to take. In the near future, my vision is to have a Virtual Center that will reach people who have had a brain injury regardless of **where they live, the severity of their injury,** or the number of years post injury. One of my goals is that everyone has access to the best experts for their case to advise on how to achieve the highest level of mental and life productivity. This level of access may be achievable through technological advances in the next few years.

Brain injury is deeply bothersome because it involves extraordinary misery juxtaposed with a *tremendous unrealized potential for brain repair.* Unfortunately, this potential is typically untapped. Think of the boon to brainomics if we significantly reduce the costs of the number one cause of disability in our country. One of the most productive ways to reduce costs from brain injuries is to prevent them altogether. Brain injury is one of the few preventable catastrophic epidemics. Prevention and restoring brainpower are achievable.

Know Brainers

1. A concussion is a brain injury.
2. The frontal lobe is the most vulnerable brain region in brain injury.
3. A brain must be allowed to recover after a concussion to achieve the highest level and long-lasting recovery.

CHAPTER 12

STAVE OFF DECLINE IN ALZHEIMER'S

I am hungry for the life that is being taken away from me through misper-ception of my abilities. I am a human being. I still exist. I have a family. I hunger for friendship, happiness, and the touch of a loved hand. What I ask for is that what is left of my life shall have meaning. Give me some-thing to live for! Help me to be strong and free until my last day.

—Unknown person with Alzheimer's

How do you know if it is normal brain glitches or something more worrisome?

Is cognitive and intellectual stimulation protective against dementia in general?

What are the advantages of early detection, since getting bad news without a cure can be devastating?

How can the rate of cognitive decline be slowed down in a progressive brain disease?

Is Alzheimer's the same in men and women?

Does keeping a person with dementia mentally engaged help or frustrate them?

The public and personal image of Alzheimer's disease is a devastating one. It conjures up awful possibilities:

- It steals your identity, your sense of self, your memories, and your ability to experience joy.
- It abducts your ability to think and recognize those you love.

Alzheimer's is a major brain disease that is viewed in the end stage at the very time of diagnosis. After a diagnosis, it is common to focus even more on diminishing abilities and what can no longer be performed rather than reframe abilities to appreciate the things that are still possible, perhaps with a little assistance or initial help. Individuals are often humiliated by the diagnosis because they think they will embarrass themselves or someone else due to being too forgetful. *Preserved abilities become obscured and ignored,* and the whole family begins to cease the lives they once lived.

And yet it is individuals diagnosed with Alzheimer's who taught me profound lessons of the brain and changed my career forever. I still remember the day I met Dave Fox. He walked into my office unannounced, without an appointment. He had been there several weeks before when he'd visited one of my team members. David had undergone comprehensive assessments by a neurologist, a neuropsychologist, a brain imaging expert, a cognitive neuroscientist, a speech-language pathologist, and a psychiatrist in an attempt to find the root cause of his increasing struggles with word finding.

Now in his early sixties, Mr. Fox was a bigger-than-life gentleman whose list of civic, business, and political accomplishments could fill a book. He was chair of the National Republican convention, a county judge, one of the largest home builders in the nation, the first major inner-city developer in a large metroplex, and he even rebuilt the State Fair of Texas. But today, he was coming to discuss a problem. He told me that he had just been diagnosed with Alzheimer's and needed my help.

My eyes got as big as saucers as I tried to think how to help this hero of my city deal with such a dreaded, horrific disease. But I said exactly what I was thinking—that I didn't know how I could help him—and explained that Alzheimer's is a progressive brain disease and that there was nothing we could do to make him better beyond the medications he'd been prescribed.

But he went on to say that our

> Alzheimer's is regarded as a disease without hope. But we have found hope in the midst of this devastating illness.

institution helps people with brain problems and since his brain was still working, there must be something we could do. Never before had I thought of a progressive brain disorder as a disease I could slow or halt, much less improve his brain fuction.

Years earlier I had reluctantly added Alzheimer's disease to my research domains to identify the similarities and differences between cognitively healthy older adults and those in the early stage of this disease.[1-3] I was hesitant because I didn't think I could handle working with individuals with relentless cognitive decline. *I had specifically chosen a field of cognitive brain health in which I could discover ways to strengthen brain capacity rather than watch it disappear. I did not want to go down a hopeless path.*

But on this day Dave Fox changed my perspective on brain health forever. I teamed up with one of my graduate students and worked with Dave for the next three to four years. The three of us made a significant impact on his ability to remain intimately engaged in his life's work longer. He was able to work through and achieve daily goals in the midst of severe word finding problems, major memory deficits, and other complex thinking problems. He inspired many professionals to rethink dementia—especially me. He motivated me to seek grant funding to systematically address whether and how much we could stave off cognitive decline to maintain daily function and quality of life in people with progressive brain disease.

Working with adults with dementia has been one of the most inspiring experiences of my life. **I have learned more about the positive possibilities from people with Alzheimer's disease than from any textbook or article I've read.** Instead of focusing on the limitations, I can now choose to focus on what can be done to cognitively stimulate those diagnosed with Alzheimer's.

Alzheimer's Disease: The Basics

Alzheimer's is the most common form of dementia, a general term for memory loss and other intellectual abilities serious enough to interfere with daily life. Alzheimer's is a progressive disease, meaning that the dementia symptoms gradually worsen over a number of years. In its early stages memory loss is mild, but in the later stages individuals lose the ability to carry on conversations and respond to their environment. Those with Alzheimer's live an average of eight years after their symptoms become noticeable to others, but survival can range from four to twenty years, depending on age and other health conditions.

> Alzheimer's is the sixth leading cause of death in the United States.

> Alzheimer's disease accounts for 50 to 80 percent of dementia cases.

Alzheimer's is not a normal part of aging, but the majority of people with Alzheimer's disease are sixty-five and older. However, dementia and Alzheimer's disease are not always diseases of the elderly. One in ten people diagnosed with Alzheimer's disease is younger than sixty-five. Some cases have been diagnosed in patients as young as their midtwenties and early thirties.[4]

Brainomics of Alzheimer's and Related Dementias

Alzheimer's is one of the **world's** fastest growing diseases. Millions more have other types of dementia, which refers to brain disorders that cause visible worsening forgetfulness, deteriorating behavioral changes, and progressively more decision-making errors.

As the Thinker generation is aging, they are voicing greater concern over memory problems than cancer and worry about what these memory problems could signify later on down the road (chapter 9). Treatable versus untreatable cognitive decline is one of the most widely shared and feared public health concerns today.

Alzheimer's has a wide-ranging impact on an individual's functionality and quality of life, and it dramatically burdens both families and whole societal infrastructures—emotionally and economically. **Some have estimated that if we can stave off the onset of dementia by two years, it will reduce the prevalence by an estimated 50 percent,** since Alzheimer's is a disease of aging. Just think of the major cost savings.

> Estimates indicate that Alzheimer's disease, a leading cause of cognitive impairment in older adults, will afflict fifteen million Americans by midcentury.

According to the Alzheimer's Association, the average lifetime cost per patient is $174,000.[5] Those dollars quickly add up, with an overall cost of health care, long-term care, and hospice estimates to be $200 billion in 2012. Projected costs for 2050 are at a record $1.1 trillion.

Since there are presently no cures for Alzheimer's disease, how do we stave off dementia? In chapter 3, we discussed the importance of getting a BrainHealth Physical for healthy people to detect early vulnerabilities so that these areas can be regained and re-wired and intact areas can be strengthened to maintain cognitive wellness. This is what we call staving off—avoiding unnecessary and preventable decline. In irreversible dementias, all the active cognitive stimulation in the world will not prevent the disease. We just want to try to take advantage of the cognitive capacity that remains as long as possible. In that sense, we should try to discover ways to:

> In 2010, nearly $203 billion was spent to care for individuals with Alzheimer's disease and other dementias.

- Forestall or thwart
- Slow the rate
- Avoid or fend off

Why Early Detection Is Important

Everyone is worried about memory loss and what it means. Currently, Alzheimer's treatment options are most effective when initiated sooner rather than later. Medical professionals and researchers refer to this early stage as mild cognitive impairment. Individuals with mild cognitive decline include those with minor memory problems, those who experience difficulty extracting the core message of conversations or reading material, or those who see changes in complex decision making.

Alzheimer's can be very frustrating for both the person and his significant other. This is especially true when you have a seemingly meaningful and co-

> Worrying does nothing more than add to the fear.

herent conversation either in person or on the phone, only for the person with dementia not to recollect an important idea an hour later. I know one man with Alzheimer's told me that his spouse was very demeaning and "lost it" by yelling at him. When I asked him how he was coping with the public display of frustration, he poignantly said, "I cannot blame her. It's not her or me that's the problem. **It's the disease that is the perpetrator.** It doesn't hurt me as I know she's raging at the disease—so am I." This is another message of wisdom from a person with moderate Alzheimer's who demonstrates intact cognitive capacity.

> The disease is the perpetrator!

Changing the Conversation About Dementia

Our genes are certainly a factor in the development of Alzheimer's, but we also play a major role in the healthy habits we adopt or ignore. Extant evidence points to the benefits of continued education, exercise, staying mentally active, and maintaining strong social ties in staving off symptoms of dementia.[6-8] Whereas there is **considerable controversy as to the benefits of available medications for Alzheimer's, strong evidence supports the view that adults should adopt lifelong habits of engaging in mentally and physically challenging activities to help the brain resist dementia to the largest degree possible.** Even if the gains are small for some, there is no downside; not to mention the additional bonus that actively engaged lifestyles mitigate loneliness and depression.

More than a decade ago, I set out to scientifically validate whether individuals with early to moderate stages of Alzheimer's could benefit from active mental stimulation when coupled with a commonly prescribed drug for the disease. The trial included individuals with confirmed diagnoses of Alzheimer's who were randomly assigned to either a group receiving mental stimulation plus drugs or to a group just taking the drug alone.

> We cannot choose our future but we can choose our habits. Our habits define our future. Choose brain-healthy habits wisely.

My results revealed a ***slower rate of decline*** in communication, functional ability, and emotional well-being in those individuals who received both mental stimulation and pharmacological intervention as compared to the drug-only group.[9] Those who were randomly selected to receive mental stimulation showed less apathy and irritability and improved quality of life.

This was one of the first studies to suggest that active mental stimulation could be a factor to exploit to maintain or potentially slow the rate of decline in early stages of progressive brain disease.

Patients with Alzheimer's rarely receive treatments or strategies beyond medication. The benefits from medication alone have not been overwhelming. Some outcomes may have negative effects or even show adverse effects. It seems that at our current state of knowledge, we should be paying attention to combined treatments of pharmacology with just as strong attention to lifestyle factors such as exercise and diet as related to cardiovascular health as well as staying cognitively active.

> It is amazing that we can neuroengineer our brains by choosing habits that use our minds even in the midst of a progressive brain disease.

As at every stage of my research career, I continuously learn the most meaningful lessons from the individuals whose lives constantly inspire my work. One individual with early-onset dementia who was younger than sixty-five advised me:

> You know what the worst part of AD is? That people have a predisposition to make certain assumptions and prejudices about me now that I have been diagnosed with Alzheimer's. It is as though diagnosis and dementedness is a single event. My common failings that would be readily dismissed in "normal" people are now given intense scrutiny, given new meanings, and are assigned new values— all of which feel dehumanizing. If I had a stroke, people wouldn't get mad if I couldn't move my arm. When I cannot remember, everyone seems to get down on me—especially me.

If medical treatments extend a terminal cancer patient's life by one or even two years, the achievement is fully celebrated. I know this because my first husband survived only six months after being diagnosed with leukemia. I would have given anything for another year or two. The potential to extend brain capacity by one year or perhaps two by active mental stimulation plus medication in Alzheimer's should be embraced as a similarly major achievement for individuals and their loved ones. These efforts can be implemented now to improve lives and to complement the major efforts to find improved vaccines or pharmacological or genetic treatments for later generations.

Stark Club for Young-Age Onset Dementia

My team and I realized that lives could be dramatically changed for the better when hope is instilled, backed by scientific research. The evidence from the cognitive training trial motivated our researchers to expand efforts in Alzheimer's disease and related dementias and launch the Stark Club, a support group for those diagnosed with Alzheimer's and their families. Named for one of the founding members, Temple Stark, this club has grown to more than fifty members over its seven years of operation. They have forged new ground as spokespersons for Alzheimer's with a steadfast determination to change attitudes about the disease and those afflicted with it.

In Audette Rackley's heartwarming book, *I Can Still Laugh,* positive changes were documented as the group members participated in an intervention program.[10] The training taught a number of ways those with Alzheimer's disease could still participate in the activities they valued while helping others at the same time. One clearly learned life message was that most individuals with Alzheimer's, given the opportunity, share the same desire as those without the disease: they longed to continue to contribute to life in meaningful ways.

> "The disease is NOT the culprit that robs us of who we are but the people around us who shun or diminish us by their pity." — Bill Tuel, Stark Club member

"We're not sitting around waiting for life to end, we're finding ways to bring more to it."

Whereas many felt wounded at the time of the diagnosis, Stark Club members found a deeper meaning in life, more than they ever expected. Focusing on using their abilities, Stark Club members volunteered in a variety of activities, including reading to children in a Head Start program, building wheelchair ramps for people's homes, delivering Meals on Wheels, serving as nursing home ombudsmen, stocking a food pantry, and serving as greeters at a senior center.

Believing that the sum of the parts was greater than the whole, under the leadership of Audette Rackley, the Stark Club undertook writing a book to share the lessons they learned. They hoped to inspire others to keep their brain edge in the midst of a diagnosis. Since being involuntarily drafted into the fight with Alzheimer's disease and other dementias, the club members knew strategies to deal with combating and overcoming the battle scars of dementia.

Pearls of Wisdom from the Stark Club

The Stark Club members and their caregivers immortalized their positive experiences in dealing with dementia, providing real-life illustrations on how not to become overwhelmed by desolate despair upon learning of the diagnosis. Here are a few pearls of wisdom from the Stark Club that are more completely conveyed in their book:

- **"Tune into changes in memory and functioning and don't just write things off."** Bill Tuel never failed at anything, but at age sixty he began having difficulty at work. As a solutions architect for a Fortune 500 company, his work required high-level mental abilities, and he was now having problems doing a job in which he'd typically excelled. He struggled to solve high-level business problems and give client presentations. Even routine tasks were becoming intermittently difficult. Doctors felt his problems were due to stress. The last thing on anyone's mind was Alzheimer's disease. Bill and his wife, Carol, learned firsthand the importance of early diagnosis; the relief of knowing what they were facing overshadowed the devastation of learning he had Alzheimer's.

- **"The spirit can still soar though abilities may be changing."** You've never met an optimist until you've met Bob Eshbaugh. His smile and warmth is evident though semantic dementia, a form of frontotemporal dementia that has affected his ability to express himself. His wife, Marie, tells a story she heard some time ago that she thinks captures Bob's spirit. As the story goes, there was a cave that only knew darkness. One day the sunshine invited the cave to come out and see its light. The cave enjoyed his day in the sun so much that he wanted to return the favor. He decided to invite the sun to come into his cave and see the darkness. The sun entered the cave, and wondered aloud, "But where's the darkness?" As Marie told the story, she said, "That's what I've learned from Bob. His approach to life is to get up in the morning and do what needs to be done that day. I've learned a lot from him in my life . . . and I'm still learning."

- **"Appreciate the simple things in life and remember every day is a gift."** Dawn and Stan Fedyniak and their daughter were devastated when they heard the diagnosis of Alzheimer's disease. Stan, a proud man, emigrated to the United States from Poland and proudly served in the United States Marines during Vietnam. He loved being an American and valued the closeness of his family. Dawn reflects, "Getting the diagnosis was so hard, but it seems we appreciate things like we never did before. Now we talk about the little details of the day and appreciate our time together more than ever. It reminds me that every day is a gift we should embrace."

The Stark Club members, their spouses, and families agree that a diagnosis of Alzheimer's disease, or other dementia, was the most challenging life event they had experienced to date; but they found resilience as they learned how to deal with new challenges. Do not get me wrong; they would quickly tell you that it was not an easy or desired life path. But being part of an active stimulation group—the Stark Club—changed their life course by helping them discover they could keep their minds active and even give back to others and not be just victims of the disease.

In the words of one of the caregivers, **"We're all looking for our purpose in life,** and our challenge is to accept our current circumstance as our purpose. When I remember that, it gives me peace. It's important to hear a message of hope and remember what really matters." Every lifetime offers countless opportunities to become more whole or to be torn to pieces. Most members of the Stark Club have now passed away, but they left us a lasting legacy by sharing their stories to give inspiration and courage for others to embrace life and therein find joy in the midst of a dreaded disease.

How Early to Seek Brain Training

As I mentioned in early chapters, keeping a brain-health fitness regime in place matters at every stage of life. It is of paramount importance that we have a benchmark against which to identify cognitive slippage and losses as early as possible. Early detection and aggressive treatment are critical to slow the rate of decline and hopefully stave off dementia in a large percentage of cases.

> 10–15 percent of individuals with mild cognitive loss go on to develop Alzheimer's each year.

Even getting a diagnosis early may help to position the person in a more positive light. When one of the Center for BrainHealth's dearest friends brought her mom to our center, she said:

> I have observed decline for the past few years. My mom is very smart and can still do almost everything, but I am worried that something is going on and it is getting to her. She is different. But whatever you find out, I warn you, you cannot tell her she has Alzheimer's disease. That news would devastate her.

Unfortunately, after all the assessments were done and her mom had seen my team and a neurologist, the news was what she had most dreaded. We told her that her memory problems were likely due to Alzheimer's disease. Although she received a painful diagnosis, her mom lived out the rest of her years with dignity and a sense of humor and style.

It is never too late or too soon to close the gap between what you could achieve and the level you are currently performing cognitively. I am actively researching the most informative and less concerning symptoms of mild cognitive loss and testing the effect of brain training to forge a meaningful brain health buffer to slow or even stop cognitive deterioration.

I am also examining how brains can be changed if brain training is given to at-risk adults. The goal is to follow individuals and see who is able to take a more positive course and who goes on to develop dementia. We are interested in using brain imaging to reveal differences in those who respond or fail to respond to treatments whether cognitive, physical exercise, pharmacological, or some combination. Cognitive decline can be improved in many, and we want to reach the most people possible.

Steps to Stave off Decline in Alzheimer's

Pursuing ways to continually engage brain stimulation and frontal lobe activity in particular is not the only tack to stave off Alzheimer's disease. Of all the clinical recommendations for preserving cognitive function, one habit that regularly comes out a winner is physical exercise. In a randomized control study of adults age fifty and older who had subjective complaints of memory problems, those who engaged in physical exercise showed gains across the board. They showed significantly higher global cognitive scores, better delayed memory scores, and less depression as compared to a control group who were provided healthy guidelines.

> Lifestyle habits may be our best option for reaching our maximum cognitive potential. Do not overlook their tremendous promise in healthy brain function.

Research on the benefits of physical exercise show comprehensive gains in increased brain blood flow in the hippocampus region[11-13] (the area supporting memory function), increased brain volume, improved delayed memory scores, and improved physical fitness as measured by VO2 max, a measure of maximum lung capacity. All of these gains potentially impact patients with any stage of dementia.

How to help a loved one diagnosed with Alzheimer's disease

When diagnosed with Alzheimer's, most fast forward and only consider the negative, but it is also important to remember that this does not necessarily mean a complete halt to life as you once knew it. It is vital to keep the brain active in areas of preserved cognitive function to slow cognitive changes.

When you see somebody with Alzheimer's disease very anxious or agitated, it's typically because they are in an environment that is either over- or understimulating. Figuring out the optimal cognitive level at which the person with Alzheimer's is currently functioning will help to set appropriate tasks and responsibilities for them. The tasks need to be somewhat challenging to keep them motivated. I recommend the following to stave off decline and maintain the built-up cognitive reserves in the earliest stages of dementia:

- Keep working as long as possible, which may in fact be years and not months and days, since we are diagnosing earlier and earlier.
- Nonetheless, once diagnosed, check out long-term disability coverage to make sure you do not lose much-needed benefits in case of job loss.
- Capitalize and highlight strengths.
- Delegate to supportive individual areas where the greatest vulnerabilities exist, such as moment-to-moment memory.
- Be sensitive to good and bad days; there is fluctuation in all brain diseases, so go with the flow. On good days, do more; on bad days, rest and avoid overly stimulating environments.
- Organize valuables, such as keys and wallet, so that they are always in the same place in order to avoid the frustration of constant treasure hunts.
- Write down or ask others to write down key information and appointments you need to know about in ONE place. Write enough to know what the time or name means.
- Tune in to minimize and avoid anxiety-producing situations.

- Do not try to do everything you were doing before; do less and you will do it better.
- Have communication with one person at a time, in a calm environment.
- Reduce distractions to the largest degree possible, since they merely add to the confusion.
- Don't hide. It takes a lot of energy to keep a diagnosis a secret. You don't have to tell everyone, but being honest with family and friends will relieve a lot of pressure and help you focus on engaging in life.
- Appreciate today. Enjoy what you have today instead of borrowing trouble from tomorrow. What you worry about may never happen and you'll have a better quality of life if you focus on what you can do now.
- Find other people with similar challenges for support. A network of people you can relate to helps, with one caveat: it is important to surround yourself with positive people.

Here are a few tips to stimulate the brain and maximize independence without pushing your loved ones past what the disease allows in more advanced disease stages:

1. **Have conversations, but give context.** Don't say, "We just talked about that," or, "Remember when?" Instead, give context. "Last year we went on a picnic at the beach . . . ." Memories will start to come together.
2. **Bring the person your dilemmas.** Ask, "What do you think about . . . ?" or, "What would you do?" People with Alzheimer's retain their wisdom during the early and moderate stages. They love to share it, and doing so helps their sense of integrity.
3. **Keep up hobbies.** The things they were good at before Alzheimer's are typically the things they'll be best at with Alzheimer's.
4. **Help them start tasks.** Getting started on everyday activities like eating and getting dressed is so hard for people with Alzheimer's. Their brains may preclude them from

initiating the first steps. But if you get them started, they will likely be able to take the next steps and even complete the task.

5. **Do activities that maintain dignity.** Watch old movies, talk about experiences or vacations, and look at pictures. It is humiliating to see a person with Alzheimer's doing childish crafts, like making bunnies out of cotton balls. It is not just about keeping busy; it's about being treated with dignity.

6. **Keep them involved.** Have them be part of conversations but do NOT talk for them. Give them time to respond and don't make it a question. Statements that provide context are easier to connect ideas to for people with Alzheimer's than answering a question.

7. **Celebrate the person.** Instead of focusing on what is impaired, focus on what the individual enjoys and can still do.

8. **Be involved, but don't take over.** Often friends and family members of those diagnosed with Alzheimer's think they must immediately jump in and control the patient's life. That's simply not the case. Be involved and willing to help, but make changes one step at a time.

9. **Try to live life as normally as possible.** Often individuals and families who are dealing with a diagnosis of Alzheimer's pull back and drastically change how they live. Instead, it is important to stay engaged in activities and relationships. Instead of stopping an activity when it starts to become too difficult, find ways to help modify it so your family member/friend can stay engaged.

Think about what is preserved even in the midst of a progressive brain disease. So much remains that these people can still do. We can transform the way we view Alzheimer's and bring life back.

For those with Alzheimer's disease and their families, the diagnosis doesn't have to mean the end of productivity and quality of life. Much can be done after receiving a heartbreaking diagnosis. Lives can be dramatically changed for the better when hope is instilled, backed by scientific research, where before it had been vanquished.

Inspired by Dave Fox and others like him, my goal is to provide hope for those who have been diagnosed with the devastating disease of Alzheimer's—hope for maintaining as much of a normal life as possible, for people with the disease as well as their caregivers; hope for finding early indicators of the disease, and hope that our research will lead to a better **understanding** of Alzheimer's and other dementias, **protection** of cognitive function, and **healing** of the brain.

Know Brainers

1. Age itself is not the cause of mental decline enough to detrimentally impact everyday life functionality.
2. Our passions are what keep us mentally thriving, even in dementia.
3. Building cognitive reserves throughout life will be a major factor in pushing out the symptoms of dementia—not to mention they are relatively inexpensive to do.
4. Active mental stimulation at a level just above the person's cognitive function can slow cognitive loss, increase connectedness, and decrease anxiety and agitation.
5. Physical exercise can help to reduce agitation and depression and potentially slow the rate of cognitive decline in those with Alzheimer's.
6. Failing to get a diagnosis and ignoring the potential onset of Alzheimer's can place increased pressure and stress on a person with the disease to overwork his or her capacity to use strategies to try to camouflage the deficits.
7. Talking about the disease once diagnosed, rather than dancing around the elephant in the room, helps all involved.

SECTION V

FULFILL THE PROMISE

CHAPTER 13

FORGE A BLAZING TRAIL OR GO BACKWARD

Your brain never stops developing and changing. It's been doing it from the time you were an embryo, and will keep doing it all your life. And this ability, perhaps, represents its greatest strength.

—James Trefil, physicist and author

Achieving your current level of human performance **starts** with your brain.

Ultimate human performance **starts and ends with YOU.** Your level of commitment can optimize your brain's cognitive capacity. Every day you wait is a gamble with diminishing returns. **Your brain performance does not stand still—it either declines or improves.** The direction depends on you—the way and degree to which you challenge your core frontal lobe brainpowers. I know that you are not likely achieving your maximal cognitive potential. What brain value are you willing to lose this year? Or will you take the necessary steps to experience brain gain?

The Promise

My goal in this book was to deliver a promise. A promise that you learn to:

- Increase your intellectual capital
- Enhance your brainpower

- Build cognitive reserves
- Slow brain slippage

It is up to you to make these promises real. The assurances will not develop just by passively reading this book with wishful thinking, but by your efforts in taking immediate and continual actions. **You control the destiny of your human cognitive performance.** You can take countless steps forward instead of going backward. However, your brain gains will not come from simply knowing what to do; they will only come when you rigorously practice strategies to build the three core frontal lobe processes:

1. Strategic attention
2. Integrated reasoning
3. Innovation

Preventing brain decline is all about everyday healthy brain habits and healthy living. You are likely your own greatest stumbling block—letting your brain edge get dull. Instead of fulfilling the promise, are you:

- adopting unhealthy mind-stressing routines that do not optimize efficient brain performance, such as chronic multitasking or shallow downloading of massive amounts of new information in the belief that more and faster will make you smarter?
- waiting for a quick fix—a pill that will make you smarter, not a continual practice of deeper, more innovative thinking?
- falsely believing in the now debunked conventional wisdom that your basic thinking capacity is unchangeable? You still hear the old tapes of an early label that you were average or not smart enough to become_____ (you fill in the blank), and you have not challenged the wrong labeling or recognized that **no one but you can limit your potential.**

You are likely to live to be ninety and older. But will your brain span match your life span? We have been working off the wrong blueprint—thinking our brains would keep going strong even though we let them become mental couch potatoes or that working our brains harder will make us smarter. We are working our brains so hard that they are fatigued, burned out, and begging for mercy. Closing the gap depends on you. The greater effort you commit to reducing the gap, the greater the increase in brainomics—the high returns from brain gain.

If you want to become better at anything, what do you do? You practice over and over. There is nothing you cannot get better at with intensive workouts. By adopting the evidence-based guide spelled out in chapters 4, 5, and 6, your brain's capacity and human performance will be rekindled, reconfigured, reshaped, and reinvigorated—no matter your age. Starting at a high level rather than an elementary one will more fully engage the complex capacity of your frontal lobe. You will become a better problem solver and decision maker when you begin to practice synthesizing big ideas and embrace the capacity of your brain to think:

- Broadly
- Strategically
- Tactically
- In a focused manner
- Innovatively
- In a more integrated way

Everyone is smart and can be smarter. You have the potential to improve your personal cognitive performance—your greatest asset and utmost gift. For sure, the major lessons about the tremendous potential of the human mind come largely from those who have participated in my research. I have witnessed significant improvements in high performers and low performers. The shared ingredient is not the baseline level of performance, but a steadfast commitment to engaging in and exercising complex cognitive thinking patterns—continually.

Take elite military personnel. I have learned monumental lessons from these high performers who participated in my brain-training research. Without exception, every member of my BrainHealth training team was inspired by the dedication of retired service members such as Navy SEALs. They are not only dedicated to putting their life on the line to defend our freedom but, just as important, they are devoted to being in the best physical and mental shape at all times. Allowing slippage is not acceptable. As a group they display an extraordinary dedication to whole body fitness and welcome the opportunity to add promising brain training to their toolbox of high performance training.

Previously the majority of the investments were made in building and restoring their amazing physical fitness. With their partnership, a goal of mine is to add the optimization of their natural intellect to the training regimen. It is a know-brainer. As one clearly commented, "When we pull a hamstring, tear a muscle, or break a bone, we undergo intensive training to regain our strength and highest human motor performance level. We never stop training. The brain is like a muscle you use in your everyday life, so why wouldn't we work even harder to escalate our brain's performance potential?"

By learning and continuously adopting the nine brain power strategies outlined in this chapter, you, too, just like the elite military professionals I have worked with, will engage in an efficient process for:

1. new learning,
2. content absorption,
3. project design and implementation,
4. problem solving,
5. breakthrough thinking, and
6. sound decision making.

Will you make and receive the greatest return on investment or will you go backward? You have nothing to lose and everything to gain by trying these methods. This book focuses on your most important and valuable natural resource—your brainpower. **What will your brain habits become now that you have read this book? Test the science for yourself and see if in fact you can become smarter this next year. Your brain potential is limitless.**

It will not be enough to pick and choose which of these processes you build. As illustrated in the diagram on page 247, all three cognitive domains provide a process to continually employ synergistically to help you think smarter—not harder.

STRATEGIC THINKING
Learning to think smarter, not harder.

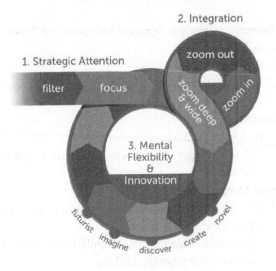

Quick Reference to the Nine Brainpowers Discussed in This Book:

Strategic Attention—Manage Brainpower

- **Brainpower of None**
  - * Take advantage of silence to think deeply and solve tough problems.

    When you hit a wall mentally, quiet your mind to regain brain energy and find fresh solutions.
- **Brainpower of One**
  - * Perform one task at a time even if for short intervals.

    Sequential task instead of multitask.
- **Brainpower of Two**
  - * Isolate and escalate your top two daily imperatives.

    Every day, identify and dedicate the majority of prime brain time to your two most important tasks. When taking a break or needing a mental shift, fill in with your necessary, but less important, tasks. Do not let these less important priorities take over.

Integrated Reasoning—Harness Dynamic Brainpower of Zoom
- **Zoom In**
  * Be in the know.

    Get the facts; know the logistics of what knowledge is needed.
- **Zoom Out**
  * Be a strategic thinker.

    Identify bigger ideas, diverse perspectives, and global themes.
- **Zoom Deep and Wide**
  * Be a tactical thinker, knowing when to apply knowledge and when not to apply.

    Formulate broader novel applications with bold, deeper, more strategic thinking.

Innovation—Harness Brain's Imagination
- **Brainpower of Infinite**
  * Know that there are endless possibilities.

    Combine disparate ideas into a multitude of concepts, discussions, and directions.
- **Brainpower of Paradox**
  * The tenacity to not get stopped or stuck by failure is the fuel that leads to the greatest advances in creativity and innovation.

    Reflect, reframe, and learn from mistakes. Mistakes are more informative than successes.
- **Brainpower of Unknown**
  * Ask why and what if.

    Seek change, not a brain on automatic pilot. Keep your brain actively curious and leading from known to unknown.

You are the CEO of your brainpower, aka the Cognitive Entrepreneur Officer. You are in control of the ways in which you will neuroengineer your brain operations. You decide every single day if you will:

- increase your intellectual capital,
- hold it in reserve, or
- spend what you have until depleted.

Each day, ask yourself these questions:

1. Am I adding to my brain account?
2. Is the currency that I am adding of value?
3. Can I escalate my level of thinking capacity?

What you do has more influence on your potential brain growth than your genetic makeup, your gender, or your inherent smarts. Discoveries are taking place at an accelerated speed, but getting the science into practice is slow. **The evidence is compelling for you to become and remain committed to enhancing your brain's performance—today and every day.** You are the neuroengineer of this intricate machine that drives how you achieve your highest human cognitive performance.

Become an advocate, become a devoted adopter by proactively and continually engaging in complex mental thinking. Start reaping the rewards of your return on investment. Put your brain at the center of your health habits. For you, **meaningful gains in human cognitive performance are probable** outcomes of persistent efforts, not to mention strengthening your functional and structural brain networks.

You have been given the greatest gift and rich natural resource—the ability to think beyond the literal data and to make complex decisions. **Do not go backward.** Keep your brain fit to actualize your immense human cognitive capacity. The gains will be profound.

As Navy SEAL Morgan Luttrell asked in the Foreword:

How far can [you] take the ability of [your] brain if [you] actually focused on training it like [you] do [your] body?

For additional tools and tips visit makeyourbrainsmarter.com.

ACKNOWLEDGMENTS

This is a book I have long wanted to write. It is a book about harnessing the untapped potential of your brain to think smarter, longer; a book about cognitive brain health for all ages and all walks of life. As is usually the case, timing works out for the best. Many discoveries set forth in the previous chapters were not yet known or published even as recently as one year ago. That is how fast brain breakthroughs are happening.

My life's work is dedicated to maximizing human cognitive potential—always. Through the years, I have been deeply influenced and inspired by my family and friends, by my patients, by my team at the Center for BrainHealth, as well as other brilliant scientists from around the world. I face each day with renewed conviction to solve the immense challenge of enhancing brain performance for all: those who are stuck or losing ground in their intellectual capacity due to brain injury, those who have been diagnosed with brain disease, and still others who have limited their potential because of inappropriate labels or lack of knowledge that something could be done to increase their brain performance. I am thankful for those individuals who have continually revealed new lessons about the immense potential of the human mind.

For their particular roles in making this book possible, I am deeply grateful to my husband, Don Chapman, whose love and encouragement inspired me in every possible way to write this book; to my son, Noah Chapman, who always worried about whether I was burning out my brain by working so hard; to my sisters Shelia Schlosberg, who was instrumental in the formation of the Center for BrainHealth, and Sue McCart, who constantly encourages me and always adds a touch of humor. I am indebted to the amazing mind and spirit of Shelly Kirkland, who worked tirelessly editing our book. I am immensely thankful to Dr. John Hart, Debbie Francis, Sarah Schoellkopf, Jennifer Zientz, Audette Rackley, Molly Keebler, Jacque Gamino, Lori Cook, Raksha Mudar, Rebecca Peterson, and every scientist and research clinician at the Center for BrainHealth at The University of Texas at Dallas who has taken on the important work of translating brain health discovery to improving lives today. A thank-you is owed to Claire Gardner for her help gathering and compiling the necessary scientific references made within these pages.

Those close to me know that my deceased husband, Carroll Bond, played a major role in my steadfast pursuit of life-changing work, making me promise before his death to finish my doctorate and someday have a center focused on helping others. I am grateful to Dr. Hanna Ulatowska, my mentor, who taught me to see the lastingness of the aging mind through scientific study.

I owe a debt of gratitude to Jan Miller Rich and Nena Madonia at Dupree Miller & Associates for their insightful guidance and tenacity in taking this project to the best publishing partner, Dominick Anfuso, along with Sydney Tanigawa at Free Press. I would be remiss in not thanking Debbie Dunlop, who instantly went to work on introducing me to Jan when she learned about the vision for this book.

In closing, I especially want to thank our brave men and women who give their lives courageously fighting for our freedom and aspire to achieve the highest brain performance possible to become the next greatest generation. I am grateful for their encouragement to expand my vision for brain health.

NOTES

Introduction

1. Jaeggi, S. M., M. Buschkuehl, J. Jonides, and W. J. Perrig. 2008. "Improving fluid intelligence with training on working memory." Proceedings of the National Academy of Sciences of the United States of America 105(19): 6829–33.

2. Sternberg, R. J. 2008. "Increasing fluid intelligence is possible after all." Proceedings of the National Academy of Sciences of the United States of America 105(19): 6791–92.

3. Diamond, A. and K. Lee. 2011. "Interventions shown to aid executive function development in children 4 to 12 years old." Science 333(6045): 959–64.

4. Kuszewski, A. 2011. "You can increase your intelligence: 5 ways to maximize your cognitive potential." "Guest Blog," Scientific American.

5. Preusse, F., E. Van der Meer, G. Deshpande, F. Krueger, and I. Wartenburger. 2011. "Fluid intelligence allows flexible recruitment of the parieto-frontal network in analogical reasoning." Frontiers in Human Neuroscience 5(22).

6. Ramsden, S., F. M. Richardson, G. Josse, M. S. C. Thomas, C. Ellis, C. Shakeshaft, M. L. Seghier, and C. J. Price. 2011. "Verbal and non-verbal intelligence changes in the teenage brain." Nature 479(7371): 113–16.

7. Wilson, R. S., E. Segawa, P. A. Boyle, and D. A. Bennett. 2012. "Influence of late-life cognitive activity on cognitive health." Neurology 78(15): 1123–29.

8. Chapman, S. B., J. Zientz, M. Weiner, R. Rosenberg, W. Frawley, and M. H. Burns. 2002. "Discourse changes in early Alzheimer disease, mild cognitive impairment, and normal aging." Alzheimer Disease and Associated Disorders 16(3): 177–86.

9. Chapman, S. B., R. Anand, G. Sparks, and C. M. Cullum. 2006. "Gist distinctions in healthy cognitive aging versus mild Alzheimer's disease." *Brain Impairment* 7: 223–33.

10. Anand, R., S. B. Chapman, A. Rackley, M. Keebler, J. Zientz, and J. Hart. 2011. "Gist reasoning training in cognitively normal seniors." *International Journal of Geriatric Psychiatry* 26(9): 961–68.

11. Cook, L. G., R. DePompei, and S. B. Chapman. 2011. "Cognitive communicative challenges in TBI: Assessment and intervention in the long term." *ASHA Perspectives* 21(1): 33–42.

12. Gamino, J., S. B. Chapman, E. L. Hull, G. R. Lyon, G. R. 2010. "Effects of higher-order cognitive strategy training on gist reasoning and fact learning in adolescents." *Frontiers in Educational Psychology* 1.

13. Vas, A. K., S. B. Chapman, L. G. Cook, A. C. Elliott, and M. Keebler. 2011. "Higher-order reasoning training years after traumatic brain injury in adults." *The Journal of Head Trauma Rehabilitation* 26(3): 224–39.

14. Chapman, S. B., C. W. Cotman, H. M. Fillit, M. Gallagher, and C. H. van Dyck. 2012. "Clinical trials: New opportunities." *Journals of Gerontology Series A: Biological Sciences and Medical Sciences*: 1–13.

15. Chapman, S. B., S. Aslan, J. S. Spence, J. J. Hart, E. K. Bartz, N. Didehbani, et al. (2013). "Neural mechanisms of brain plasticity with complex cognitive training in healthy seniors." *Cerebral Cortex*. doi: 10.1093/cercor/bht234.

16. Horn, J. L. 1982. "The aging of human abilities." In B. B. Wolman, ed., *Handbook of Developmental Psychology*, pp 847–70 Englewood Cliffs, N.J.: Prentice-Hall, 1982.

17. Hanushek, E. A. and L. Woessmann. 2011. "How much do educational outcomes matter in OECD countries?" *Economic Policy* 26(67): 427–91.

18. Ulatowska, H. K., S. B. Chapman, A. P. Highly, and J. Prince. 1998. "Discourse in healthy old-elderly adults: A longitudinal study." *Aphasiology* 12(⅞): 619–33.

19. Valenzuela, M. J., M. Breakspear, and P. Sachdev. 2007. "Complex mental activity and the aging brain: Molecular, cellular and cortical network mechanisms." *Brain Research Reviews* 56(1): 198–213.

20. Anand, R., S. B. Chapman, A. Rackley, and J. Zientz. 2011. "Brain health fitness: Beyond retirement." *Educational Gerontology, International Journal* 37(6): 450–66.

21. Anand, R., M. A. Motes, M. J. Maguire, P. S. Moore, S. B. Chapman, and J. Hart. 2009. "Neural basis of abstracted meaning." *Neurobiology of Language*, Chicago, IL.

22. Roldan-Tapia, L., J. Garcia, R. Canovas, and I. Leon. 2012. "Cognitive re-

serve, age, and their relation to attentional and executive functions." *Applied Neuropsychology* 19(1): 2–8.

Section I: Discover the Frontal Lobe Frontier
Chapter 1 Your Brain, Your Productivity

1. Anand, R., S. B. Chapman, A. Rackley, M. Keebler, J. Zientz, and J. Hart. 2011. "Gist reasoning training in cognitively normal seniors." *International Journal of Geriatric Psychiatry* 26(9): 961–68.

2. Gamino, J., S. B. Chapman, E. L. Hull, G. R. Lyon. 2010. "Effects of higher-order cognitive strategy training on gist reasoning and fact learning in adolescents." *Frontiers in Educational Psychology* 1.

3. Roldan-Tapia, L., J. Garcia, R. Canovas, and I. Leon. 2012. "Cognitive reserve, age, and their relation to attentional and executive functions." *Applied Neuropsychology* 19(1): 2–8.

4. Chapman, S. B., C. W. Cotman, H. M. Fillit, M. Gallagher, and C. H. van Dyck. 2012. "Clinical trials: New opportunities." *Journals of Gerontology Series A: Biological Sciences and Medical Sciences*: 1–13.

5. Chapman, S. B., S. Aslan, J. S. Spence, J. J. Hart, E. K. Bartz, N. Didehbani, et al. (2013). "Neural mechanisms of brain plasticity with complex cognitive training in healthy seniors." *Cerebral Cortex*. doi: 10.1093/cercor/bht234.

6. Braver, T. S. 2012. "The variable nature of cognitive control: a dual mechanisms framework." *Trends in Cognitive Sciences* 16(2): 106–13.

7. Kruglanski, A. W., J. J. Belanger, X. Y. Chen, C. Kopetz, A. Pierro, L. Mannetti. 2012. "The energetics of motivated cognition: A force-field analysis." *Psychological Review* 119(1): 1–20.

8. Chapman et al. 2013. "Neural mechanisms of brain plasticity with complex cognitive training in healthy seniors." *Cerebral Cortex*. doi: 10.1093/cercor/bht234.

9. Valenzuela, M. J., M. Breakspear, and P. Sachdev. 2007. "Complex mental activity and the aging brain: Molecular, cellular and cortical network mechanisms." *Brain Research Reviews* 56(1): 198–213.

10. Lewis, C. M., A. Baldassarre, G. Committeri, G. L. Romani, and M. Corbetta. 2009. "Learning sculpts the spontaneous activity of the resting human brain." Proceedings of the National Academy of Sciences of the United States of America 106(41): 17558–63.

11. Greenwood, P. M., and R. Parasuraman. 2010. "Neuronal and cognitive plasticity: A neurocognitive framework for ameliorating cognitive aging." *Frontiers in Aging Neuroscience* 2: 150.

12. Seeley, W. W., V. Menon, A. F. Schatzberg, J. Keller, G. H. Glover, H. Kenna, et al. 2007. "Dissociable intrinsic connectivity networks for salience processing and executive control." *Journal of Neuroscience* 27(9): 2349–56.

13. Hanushek, E. A. and L. Woessmann. 2011. "How much do educational outcomes matter in OECD countries?" *Economic Policy* 26(67): 427–91.

14. Roldan-Tapia et al. "Cognitive reserve, age, and their relation to attentional and executive functions," 2–8.

15. Kruglanski et al. "The energetics of motivated cognition: A force-field analysis," 1–20.

16. Preusse, F., E. Van der Meer, G. Deshpande, F. Krueger, and I. Wartenburger. 2011. "Fluid intelligence allows flexible recruitment of the parieto-frontal network in analogical reasoning." *Frontiers in Human Neuroscience* 5(22).

17. Seeley et al. "Dissociable intrinsic connectivity networks for salience processing and executive control," 2349–56.

18. Badre, D. and M. D'Esposito. 2009. "Is the rostro-caudal axis of the frontal lobe hierarchical?" *Nature Reviews, Neuroscience* 10(9): 659–69.

19. Christoff, K., K. Keramantian, G. Alan, R. Smith, and B. Madler. 2009. "Prefrontal organization of cognitive control according to levels of abstraction." *Brain Research* 1286: 94–105.

20. Stuss, D. T. 2011. "Functions of the frontal lobes: Relation to executive functions." *Journal of the International Neuropsychological Society* 17(5): 759–65.

21. Collins, A. and E. Koechlin. 2012. "Reasoning, learning, and creativity: frontal lobe function and human decision-making." *PLoS Biology* 10(3): e1001293.

Chapter 2 Frontal Lobe Fitness Rules

1. Braver, T. S. 2012. "The variable nature of cognitive control: a dual mechanisms framework." *Trends in Cognitive Sciences* 16(2): 106–13.

2. Collins, A. and E. Koechlin. 2012. "Reasoning, learning, and creativity: frontal lobe function and human decision-making." *PLoS Biology* 10(3): e1001293.

3. Mozolic, J. L., A. B. Long, A. R. Morgan, M. Rawley-Payne, and P. J. Laurienti. 2011. "A cognitive training intervention improves modality-specific attention in a randomized controlled trial of healthy older adults." *Neurobiology of Aging* 32(4): 655–68.

4. Gogtay, N., J. N. Giedd, L. Lusk, K. M. Hayashi, D. Greenstein, A. C. Vaituzis, et al. 2004. "Dynamic mapping of human cortical development dur-

ing childhood through early adulthood." *Proceedings of the National Academy of Sciences of the United States of America* 101(21): 8174–79.

5. Casey, B. J., N. Tottenham, C. Liston, and S. Durston. 2005. "Imaging the developing brain: What have we learned about cognitive development?" *Trends in Cognitive Science* 9(3): 104–10.

6. Diamond, A. 2011. "Biological and social influences on cognitive control processes dependent on prefrontal cortex." *Progress in Brain Research* 189: 319–39.

7. Keating, D. P. 2004. "Cognitive and brain development." In R. J. Lerner and L. D. Steinberg (Eds.), *Handbook of Adolescent Psychology* (2nd ed). Hoboken, NJ: Wiley: 45–84.

8. Badre, D. and M. D'Esposito. 2009. "Is the rostro-caudal axis of the frontal lobe hierarchical?" *Nature Reviews, Neuroscience* 10(9): 659–69.

9. Stuss, D. T. 2011. "Functions of the frontal lobes: Relation to executive functions." *Journal of the International Neuropsychological Society* 17(5): 759–65.

10. Goel, V. and R. J. Dolan. 2003. "Reciprocal neural response within lateral and ventral medial prefrontal cortex during hot and cold reasoning." *Neuro-Image* 20: 2314–21.

11. Carlile, P. R. 2004. "Transferring, translating, and transforming: An integrative framework for managing knowledge across boundaries." *Organization Science* 15(5): 555–68.

12. Jung-Beeman, M., E. M. Bowden, J. Haberman, J. L. Frymiare, S. Arambel-Liu, R. Greenblatt, et al. 2004. "Neural Activity When People Solve Verbal Problems with Insight." *PLoS Biology* 2(4): 500–510.

13. Baltes, P. B. and U. M. Staudinger. 2000. "Wisdom: A metaheuristic (pragmatic) to orchestrate mind and virtue toward excellence." *American Psychologist* 55(1): 122–36.

14. Sandku, S. and J. Bhattacharya. 2008. "Deconstructing insight: EEG correlates of insightful problem solving." *PLoS ONE* 3(1): e1459.

15. Sternberg, R. J. 2008. "Increasing fluid intelligence is possible after all." *Proceedings of the National Academy of Sciences of the United States of America* 105(19): 6791–92.

16. Norman, D. A. and T. Shallice. 1983. "Attention to action—Willed and automatic-control of behavior." *Bulletin of the Psychonomic Society* 21(5): 354.

17. Eyrolle, H. and J. M. Cellier. 2000. "The effects of interruptions in work activity: Field and laboratory results." *Applied Ergonomics* 31: 537–43.

18. Mark, G., V. M. Gonzalez, and J. Harris. 2005. "No Task Left Behind? Exam-

ining the Nature of Fragmented Work." CHI 2005 | PAPERS: Take a Number, Stand in Line (Interruptions & Attention 1): 321–30.

19. Glascher, J., D. Rudauf, R. Colom, L. K. Paul, D. Tranel, H. Damasio, and R. Adolphs. 2010. "Distributed neural system for general intelligence revealed by lesion mapping." Proceedings of the National Academy of Sciences of the United States of America 107(10): 4705–9.

20. Dreher, J-C., E. Koechlin, S. O. Ali, and J. Grafman. 2002. "The roles of timing and task order during task switching." NeuroImage 17: 95–109.

21. Kuchinskas, S. 2008. "Multitasking is a myth: Your brain is actually rapidly switching focus from one task to another." WebMD the Magazine: 1–2.

22. Kruglanski, A. W., J. J. Belanger, X. Y. Chen, C. Kopetz, A. Pierro, and L. Mannetti. 2012. "The energetics of motivated cognition: A force-field analysis." Psychological Review 119(1): 1–20.

23. Cattell, R. B. 1971. Abilities: Their Structure, Growth and Action. Boston: Houghton-Mifflin.

24. Levine, B., I. H. Robertson, L. Clare, G. Carter, J. Hong, B. A. Wilson, et al. 2000. "Rehabilitation of executive functioning: An experimental-clinical validation of goal management training." Journal of the International Neuropsychological Society, 6(3): 299–312.

25. Sternberg. "Increasing fluid intelligence is possible after all," 6791–92.

26. Lewis, C. M., A. Baldassarre, G. Committeri, G. L. Romani, and M. Corbetta. 2009. "Learning sculpts the spontaneous activity of the resting human brain." Proceedings of the National Academy of Sciences of the United States of America 106(41): 17558–63.

27. Badre and D'Esposito. "Is the rostro-caudal axis of the frontal lobe hierarchical?" 659–669.

28. Diamond. "Biological and social influences on cognitive control processes dependent on prefrontal cortex," 319–39.

29. Carlile. "Transferring, translating, and transforming: An integrative framework for managing knowledge across boundaries," 555–68.

30. Burgess, P. W., E. Veitcha, A. L. Costello, and T. Shallice. 1999. "The cognitive and neuroanatomical correlates of multitasking." Neuropsychologia 38(2000): 848–63.

31. De Kloet, E. R., M. Joels, and F. Holsboer. 2005. "Stress and the brain: From adaptation to disease." Nature Reviews, Neuroscience 6(6): 463–75.

32. Clark, K. and R. Smith. 2008. "Unleashing the Power of Design Thinking." Design Management Review Summer: 8–15.

33. Clark and Smith. "Unleashing the Power of Design Thinking," 8–15.
34. Begley, S. 2007. "New research finds some brain functions actually improve with age. Our reporter on delayed retirement and how to stay sharp." *Wall Street Journal* online, W1.
35. Scardamalia, M. and C. Bereiter. 2008. "Pedagogical biases in educational technologies." *Educational Technology* XLVIII(3): 3–11.
36. Christoff, K., K. Keramantian, G. Alan, R. Smith, and B. Madler. 2009. "Prefrontal organization of cognitive control according to levels of abstraction." *Brain Research* 1286: 94–105.
37. Stuss. "Functions of the frontal lobes: Relation to executive functions," 759–65.
38. Goel and Dolan. "Reciprocal neural response within lateral and ventral medial prefrontal cortex during hot and cold reasoning," 2314–21.
39. Glascher et al. "Distributed neural system for general intelligence revealed by lesion mapping," 4705–9.
40. Saladin, K. 2007. *Anatomy and Physiology: The Unity of Form and Function.* New York: McGraw Hill.
41. Dumitriu, D., J. Hao, Y. Hara, J. Kaufmann, W. G. M. Janssen, W. Lou, et al. 2010. "Selective changes in thin spine density and morphology in monkey prefrontal cortex correlate with aging-related cognitive impairment." *Journal of Neuroscience* 30(22): 7507–15.
42. Grossmann, I., J. Na, M. E. W. Varnum, D. C. Park, S. Kitayama and R. E. Nisbett. 2010. "Reasoning about social conflicts improves into old age." Proceedings of the National Academy of Sciences of the United States of America 107(16): 7246–50.
43. Raz, N., A. Williamson, F. Gunning-Dixon, D. Head, and J. D. Acker. 2000. "Neuroanatomical and cognitive correlates of adult age differences in acquisition of a perceptual-motor skill." *Microscopy Research and Technique* 51(1): 85–93.
44. Miller, E. K. 2000. "The prefrontal cortex and cognitive control." *Nature Reviews, Neuroscience* 3(11): 1066–68.
45. Giedd, J. N., L. S. Clasen, R. Lenroot, D. Greenstein, G. L. Wallace, S. Ordaz, et al. 2006. "Puberty-related influences on brain development." *Molecular and Cellular Endocrinology* 254–255: 154–62.
46. Diamond, A. and K. Lee. 2011. "Interventions shown to aid executive function development in children 4 to 12 years old." *Science* 333(6045): 959–64.
47. Kruglanski et al. "The energetics of motivated cognition: A force-field analysis," 1–20.

48. Kuchinskas. "Multitasking is a myth: Your brain is actually rapidly switching focus from one task to another," 1–2.

49. Burgess. "The cognitive and neuroanatomical correlates of multitasking," 848–63.

50. Ophir, E., C. Nass, and A. D. Wagner. 2009. "Cognitive control in media multitaskers." Proceedings of the National Academy of Sciences of the United States of America 106(37): 15583–87.

51. Ophir et al. "Cognitive control in media multitaskers," 15583–87.

52. Van der Linden, D., M. Frese, and T. F. Meijman. 2003. "Mental fatigue and the control of cognitive processes: effects on perseveration and planning." Acta Psychologica 113: 45–65.

53. Sternberg. "Increasing fluid intelligence is possible after all," 6791–92.

54. Valenzuela, M. J., M. Breakspear, and P. Sachdev. 2007. "Complex mental activity and the aging brain: Molecular, cellular and cortical network mechanisms." Brain Research Reviews 56(1): 198–213.

55. Begley. "New research finds some brain functions actually improve with age. Our reporter on delayed retirement and how to stay sharp," W1.

56. Gould, E., A. Beylin, P. Tanapat, A. Reeves, and T. J. Shors. 1999. "Learning enhances adult neurogenesis in the hippocampal formation." Nature Neuroscience 2(3): 260–5.

57. Gould, E., P. Tanapat, N. B. Hastings, and T. J. Shors. 1999. "Neurogenesis in adulthood: A possible role in learning." Trends in Cognitive Sciences 3(5): 186–92.

58. Cracchiolo, J. R., T. Mori, S. J. Nazian, J. Tan, H. Potter, and G. W. Arendash. 2007. "Enhanced cognitive activity—over and above social or physical activity—is required to protect Alzheimer's mice against cognitive impairment, reduce Abeta deposition, and increase synaptic immunoreactivity." Neurobiology of Learning and Memory 88: 277–94.

59. Gilkey, R. and C. Kilts. 2007. "Cognitive Fitness." Harvard Business Review: 1–9.

60. Sternberg. "Increasing fluid intelligence is possible after all," 6791–92.

61. Greenwood, P. M. and R. Parasuraman. 2010. "Neuronal and cognitive plasticity: A neurocognitive framework for ameliorating cognitive aging." Frontiers in Aging Neuroscience 2: 150.

62. Paavola, S. and K. Hakkarainen. 2005. "The knowledge creation metaphor—An emergent epistemological approach to learning." Science & Education 14: 535–57.

63. Horn, J. L. 1982. "The aging of human abilities." In *Intelligence: Measurement, Theory and Public Policy,* edited by B. B. Wolman, 29–73. Urbana: University of Illinois Press.

64. Hedden, T. and J. D. Gabrieli. 2004. "Insights into the ageing mind: a view from cognitive neuroscience." *Nature Reviews, Neuroscience* 5(2): 87–96.

65. Grady, C. L., M. V. Springer, D. Hongwanishkul, A. R. McIntosh, and G. Winocur. 2006. "Age-related changes in brain activity across the adult lifespan." *Journal of Cognitive Neuroscience* 18(2): 227–41.

66. Salthouse, T. A. 2006. "Aging of thought." In E. Bialystok and F. I. M. Craik (eds.), *Lifespan cognition: Mechanisms of change.* NY: Oxford University Press.

67. Salthouse, T. A. 2011. "Neuroanatomical substrates of age-related cognitive decline." *Psychological Bulletin* 137(5): 753–84.

68. Craik, F. M. and A. M. Schloerscheidt. 2011. "Age-related differences in recognition memory: Effects of materials and context change." *Psychology and Aging* 26(3): 671–77.

69. Lewis, C. M., A. Baldassarre, G. Committeri, G. L. Romani, and M. Corbetta. 2009. "Learning sculpts the spontaneous activity of the resting human brain." Proceedings of the National Academy of Sciences of the United States of America 106(41): 17558–63.

70. Greenwood, P. M. and R. Parasuraman. 2010. "Neuronal and cognitive plasticity: A neurocognitive framework for ameliorating cognitive aging." *Frontiers in Aging Neuroscience* 2: 150.

71. Mozolic, J. L., A. B. Long, A. R. Morgan, M. Rawley-Payne, and P. J. Laurienti. 2011. "A cognitive training intervention improves modality-specific attention in a randomized controlled trial of healthy older adults." *Neurobiology of Aging* 32(4): 655–68.

72. Ball, K., D. B. Berch, K. F. Helmers, J. B. Jobe, M. D. Leveck, M. Marsiske, et al. 2002. "Effects of cognitive training interventions with older adults: A randomized controlled trial." *Journal of the American Medical Association* 288(18): 2271–81.

73. Hartman-Stein, P. and E. Potkanowicz. 2003. "Behavioral determinants of healthy aging: Good news for the baby boomer generation." *Online Journal of Issues in Nursing* 8(2), Manuscript 5.

74. Acevedo, A. and D. A. Loewenstein. 2007. "Nonpharmacological cognitive interventions in aging and dementia." *Journal of Geriatric Psychiatry and Neurology* 20(4): 239–49.

75. Valenzuela, Breakspear, and Sachdev. "Complex mental activity and the aging brain: Molecular, cellular and cortical network mechanisms," 198–213.

76. Lewis, C. M. A. Baldassarre, G. Committeri, G. L. Romani, and M. Corbetta. 2009. "Learning sculpts the spontaneous activity of the resting human brain." Proceedings of the National Academy of Sciences of the United States of America 106(41): 17558–63.

77. Wilson, R. S., C. F. M. de Leon, L. L. Barnes, J. A. Schneider, J. L. Bienias, D. A. Evans, and D. A. Bennett. 2002. "Participation in cognitively stimulating activities and risk of incident Alzheimer disease." Journal of the American Medical Association 287(6): 742–48.

78. Ulatowska, H. K., S. B. Chapman, A. P. Highly, and J. Prince. 1998. "Discourse in healthy old-elderly adults: A longitudinal study." Aphasiology 12(⅞): 619–33.

79. Greenwood and Parasuraman. "Neuronal and cognitive plasticity: A neurocognitive framework for ameliorating cognitive aging," 150.

80. Mozolic et al. "A cognitive training intervention improves modality-specific attention in a randomized controlled trial of healthy older adults," 655–68.

81. Begley. "New research finds some brain functions actually improve with age. Our reporter on delayed retirement and how to stay sharp," W1.

82. Grossmann et al. "Reasoning about social conflicts improves into old age," 7246–50.

83. Guttman, M. 2001. "The Aging Brain." USC Health Magazine (Spring). http://www.usc.edu/hsc/info/pr/hmm/01spring/brain.html.

84. Guttman. "The Aging Brain."

85. MacMillan, M. 2000. An Odd Kind of Fame: Stones of Phineas Gage. Cambridge: MIT Press.

86. Rao, V. and C. Lyketsos. 2000. "Neuropsychiatric sequelae of traumatic brain Injury." Psychosomatics 41(2): 95–103.

87. Guskiewicz, K. M., S. W. Marshall, J. Bailes, M. McCrea, R. C. Cantu, C. Randolph, et al. 2005. "Association between recurrent concussion, mild cognitive impairment, and Alzheimer's disease in retired professional football players." Neurosurgery 57(4): 719–24.

88. Chen, A. J. W., G. M. Abrams, and M. D'Esposito. 2006. "Functional reintegration of prefrontal neural networks for enhancing recovery after brain injury." Journal of Head Trauma Rehabilitation 21(2): 107.

89. Bloss, E. B., W. G. Janssen, B. S. McEwen, and J. H. Morrison. 2010. "Interactive effects of stress and aging on structural plasticity in the prefrontal cortex." Journal of Neuroscience 30(19): 6726–31.

90. Anand, R., S. B. Chapman, A. Rackley, M. Keebler, J. Zientz, and J. Hart. 2011. "Gist reasoning training in cognitively normal seniors." *International Journal of Geriatric Psychiatry* 26(9): 961–68.

91. Gamino, J., S. B. Chapman, E. L. Hull, G. R. Lyon. 2010. "Effects of higher-order cognitive strategy training on gist reasoning and fact learning in adolescents." *Frontiers in Educational Psychology* 1.

92. Vas, A. K., S. B. Chapman, L. G. Cook, A. C. Elliott, and M. Keebler. 2011. "Higher-order reasoning training years after traumatic brain injury in adults." *The Journal of Head Trauma Rehabilitation* 26(3): 224–39.

93. Anand, R., S. B. Chapman, A. Rackley, and J. Zientz, J. 2011. "Brain health fitness: Beyond retirement." *Educational Gerontology, International Journal* 37(6): 450–66.

94. Chapman, S. B., H. K. Ulatowska, and C. Branch. 1994. "Successful aging: Depth of discourse processing and utilization of wisdom." Presentation given at the Conference of the Gerontological Society of America.

95. Kuszewski, A. 2011. "You can increase your intelligence: 5 ways to maximize your cognitive potential." *Scientific American Guest Blog*.

96. Carlile. "Transferring, translating, and transforming: An integrative framework for managing knowledge across boundaries," 555–68.

97. Levine et al. "Rehabilitation of executive functioning: An experimental-clinical validation of goal management training," 299–312.

98. Clark and Smith. "Unleashing the Power of Design Thinking," 8–15.

99. Paavola and Hakkarainen "The knowledge creation metaphor—An emergent epistemological approach to learning," 535–57.

100. Owen, A. M., A. Hampshire, J. A. Grahn, R. Stenton, S. Dajani, A. S. Burns, R. J. Howard, C. G. Ballard. 2010. "Putting brain training to the test." *Nature* 465(7299): 775–78.

101. Anand et al. "Gist reasoning training in cognitively normal seniors," 961–68.

102. Gamino, J., S. B. Chapman, E. L. Hull, G. R. Lyon. 2010. "Effects of higher-order cognitive strategy training on gist reasoning and fact learning in adolescents." *Frontiers in Educational Psychology* 1.

103. Vas et al. "Higher-order reasoning training years after traumatic brain injury in adults," 224–39.

104. Chapman, S. B., J. F. Gamino, and R. A. Mudar. 2012. "Higher order strategic gist reasoning in adolescence." In Reyna, V. F., S. B. Chapman, M. Dougherty, and J. Confrey (Eds.), *The Adolescent Brain: Learning, Reasoning, and Decision Making*. Washington, DC: American Psychological Association.

CHAPTER 3 A Checkup from Your Neck Up

1. Knickman, J. R. and E. K. Snell. 2002. "The 2030 problem: Caring for aging baby boomers." *Health Services Research* 37(4) 849–84.

2. Taubert, M., B. Draganski, A. Anwander, K. Muller, A. Horstmann, A. Villringer, and P. Ragert. 2010. "Dynamic properties of human brain structure: Learning-related changes in cortical areas and associated fiber connections." *Journal of Neuroscience* 30(35): 11670–7.

3. Vas, A. K., S. B. Chapman, L. G. Cook, A. C. Elliott, and M. Keebler. 2011. "Higher-order reasoning training years after traumatic brain injury in adults." *The Journal of Head Trauma Rehabilitation* 26(3): 224–39.

4. Seeley, W. W., V. Menon, A. F. Schatzberg, J. Keller, G. H. Glover, H. Kenna, et al. 2007. "Dissociable intrinsic connectivity networks for salience processing and executive control." *Journal of Neuroscience* 27(9): 2349–56.

5. Guskiewicz, K. M., S. W. Marshall, J. Bailes, M. McCrea, R. C. Cantu, C. Randolph, et al. 2005. "Association between recurrent concussion, mild cognitive impairment, and Alzheimer's disease in retired professional football players." *Neurosurgery* 57(4): 719–24.

6. Bassett, D. S., N. F. Wymbs, M. A. Porterc, P. J. Muchae, J. M. Carlson, and S. T. Grafton. 2011. "Dynamic reconfiguration of human brain networks during learning." Proceedings of the National Academy of Sciences of the United States of America 108(18): 7641–46.

7. Sternberg, R. J. 2008. "Increasing fluid intelligence is possible after all." Proceedings of the National Academy of Sciences of the United States of America 105(19): 6791–92.

8. Kuszewski, A. 2011. "You can increase your intelligence: 5 ways to maximize your cognitive potential." "Guest Blog," *Scientific American.*

9. Lewis, C. M., A. Baldassarre, G. Committeri, G. L. Romani, and M. Corbetta. 2009. "Learning sculpts the spontaneous activity of the resting human brain." Proceedings of the National Academy of Sciences of the United States of America 106(41): 17558–63.

10. Greenwood, P. M. and R. Parasuraman. 2010. "Neuronal and cognitive plasticity: A neurocognitive framework for ameliorating cognitive aging." *Frontiers in Aging Neuroscience* 2: 150.

11. Scardamalia, M. and C. Bereiter. 2006. "Knowledge building: Theory, pedagogy, and technology." In K. Sawyer (ed.), *Cambridge Handbook of the Learning Sciences.* New York: Cambridge University Press: 97–118.

12. Kramer, A. F. and K. I. Erickson. 2007. "Capitalizing on cortical plasticity:

Influence of physical activity on cognition and brain function." *Trends in Cognitive Sciences* 11(8): 342–48.

13. Willis, S. L., S. L. Tennstedt, M. Marsiske, K. Ball, J. Elias, K. M. Koepke, et al. 2006. "Long-term effects of cognitive training on everyday functional outcomes in older adults." *Journal of the American Medical Association* 296(23): 2805–14.

14. Sagi, Y., I. Tavor, S. Hofstetter, S. Tzur-Moryosef, T. Blumenfeld-Katzirand, and Y. Assaf. 2012. "Learning in the Fast Lane: New Insights into Neuroplasticity." *Neuron* 73(6): 1195–203.

15. Chapman, S. B., J. Zientz, M. Weiner, R. Rosenberg, W. Frawley, and M. H. Burns. 2002. "Discourse changes in early Alzheimer disease, mild cognitive impairment, and normal aging." *Alzheimer Disease and Associated Disorders* 16(3): 177–86.

16. Chapman, S. B., R. Anand, G. Sparks, and C. M. Cullum. 2006. "Gist distinctions in healthy cognitive aging versus mild Alzheimer's disease." *Brain Impairment* 7: 223–33.

17. Della Sala, S., G. Cocchini, R. H. Logie, M. Allerhand, and S. E. MacPherson. 2010. "Dual task during encoding, maintenance, and retrieval in Alzheimer's Disease." *Journal of Alzheimers Disease* 19(2): 503–15.

18. MacPherson, S. 2012. "Dual task abilities as a possible preclinical marker of Alzheimer's Disease in carriers of the E280A presenilin-1 mutation." *Journal of the International Neuropsychological Society* 18(02): 234–41.

19. Anand, R., S. B. Chapman, A. Rackley, M. Keebler, J. Zientz, and J. Hart. 2011. "Gist reasoning training in cognitively normal seniors." *International Journal of Geriatric Psychiatry* 26(9): 961–68.

20. Ulatowska, H. K., S. B. Chapman, A. P. Highly and J. Prince. 1998. "Discourse in healthy old-elderly adults: A longitudinal study." *Aphasiology* 12(⅞): 619–33.

21. Baltes, P. B. and U. M. Staudinger. 2000. "Wisdom: A metaheuristic (pragmatic) to orchestrate mind and virtue toward excellence." *American Psychologist* 55(1): 122–36.

22. Vas, Chapman, Cook et al. "Higher-order reasoning training years after traumatic brain injury in adults," 224–39.

23. Vas, A., S. B. Chapman, D. Krawczyk, K. Krishnan, and M. Keebler. 2010. "Executive control training to enhance frontal plasticity in traumatic brain injury." International Brain Injury Association's Eighth World Congress on Brain Injury, *Brain Injury* 24(3): 115–463.

24. Chapman, S. B., G. Sparks, H. S. Levin, M. Dennis, C. Roncadin, L. Zhang, and J. Song. 2004. "Discourse macrolevel processing after severe pediatric traumatic brain injury." *Developmental Neuropsychology* 25(1&2): 37–60.

25. Chapman, S. B., J. F. Gamino, L. G. Cook, G. Hanten, X. Li, and H. S. Levin. 2006. "Impaired discourse gist and working memory in children after brain injury." *Brain and Language* 97: 178–88.

26. Roldan-Tapia, L., J. Garcia, R. Canovas, and I. Leon. "Cognitive reserve, age, and their relation to attentional and executive functions." *Applied Neuropsychology* 19 (1): 2–8.

27. Foubert-Samier, A., G. Catheline, H. Amieva, B. Dilharreguy, C. Helmer, M. Allard, and J. F. Dartigues. 2010. "Education, occupation, leisure activities, and brain reserve: a population-based study." *Neurobiology of Aging* 33(2): 423e15.

28. Valenzuela, M. J., M. Breakspear, and P. Sachdev. 2007. "Complex mental activity and the aging brain: Molecular, cellular and cortical network mechanisms." *Brain Research Reviews* 56(1): 198–213.

29. Levine, B., I. H. Robertson, L. Clare, G. Carter, J. Hong, B. A. Wilson, et al. 2000. "Rehabilitation of executive functioning: An experimental-clinical validation of goal management training." *Journal of the International Neuropsychological Society* 6(3): 299–312.

30. Gilkey, R. and C. Kilts. 2007. "Cognitive Fitness." *Harvard Business Review*: 1–9.

31. Chapman, Zientz, et al. "Discourse changes in early Alzheimer disease, mild cognitive impairment, and normal aging," 177–86.

32. Chapman, Anand, et al. "Gist distinctions in healthy cognitive aging versus mild Alzheimer's disease," 223–33.

33. Cook, L. G., R. DePompei, and S. B. Chapman. 2010. "Cognitive communicative challenges in TBI: Assessment and intervention in the long term." *ASHA Perspectives, Division 2.*

34. Gamino, J., S. B. Chapman, E. L. Hull, G. R. Lyon, G. R. 2010. "Effects of higher-order cognitive strategy training on gist reasoning and fact learning in adolescents." *Frontiers in Educational Psychology* 1.

35. Vas, Chapman, Cook, et al. "Higher-order reasoning training years after traumatic brain injury in adults," 224–39.

36. Chapman, S. B., S. Aslan, J. S. Spence, J. J. Hart, E. K. Bartz, N. Didehbani, et al. (2013). "Neural mechanisms of brain plasticity with complex cognitive training in healthy seniors." *Cerebral Cortex.* doi: 10.1093/cercor/bht234.

37. Anand, R., S. B. Chapman, A. Rackley, and J. Zientz. 2011. "Brain health fitness: Beyond retirement." *Educational Gerontology, International Journal* 37(6): 450–66.

38. Chapman, S. B. and H. K. Ulatowska. 1997. "Discourse in dementia: Consideration of consciousness." In M. I. Stamenov (Ed.), *Language Structure, Discourse and the Access to Consciousness*. Philadelphia: John Benjamin Publishing Company: 155–88.

Section II Maximize Your Cognitive Performance
Chapter 4 Strengthen Your Strategic Brain Habits

1. Gamino, J., S. B. Chapman, E. L. Hull, and G. R. Lyon. 2010. "Effects of higher-order cognitive strategy training on gist reasoning and fact learning in adolescents." *Frontiers in Educational Psychology* 1.

2. Chapman, S. B., J. F. Gamino, and R. A. Mudar. 2012. "Higher order strategic gist reasoning in adolescence." In Reyna, V. F., S. B. Chapman, M. Dougherty, and J. Confrey (eds.), *The Adolescent Brain: Learning, Reasoning, and Decision Making*. Washington, DC: American Psychological Association.

3. Clark, D. 2011. "Five Things You Should Stop Doing in 2012." "HBR Blog," *Harvard Business Review.*

4. Zeldes, N., D. Sward, and S Louchheim. 2007. "Infomania: Why we can't afford to ignore it any longer." *First Monday* 12(8–6).

5. Czerwinski, M., E. Horvitz, and S. Wilhite. 2010. "A Diary Study of Task Switching and Interruptions." Microsoft Research, 1–8. http://research .microsoft.com/en-us/um/people/horvitz/taskdiary.pdf.

6. Schwartz, T. 2012. "The Magic of Doing One Thing at a Time," "HBR Blog," *Harvard Business Review.*

7. Sandku, S. and J. Bhattacharya. 2008. "Deconstructing insight: EEG correlates of insightful problem solving." *PLoS ONE* 3(1): e1459.

8. Lehrer, J. 2008. Annals of Science, "The Eureka Hunt." *The New Yorker.* 40.

9. Kounios J. and M. Beeman. 2009. "The Aha! Moment: The cognitive neuroscience of insight." *Current Directions in Psychological Science* 18: 210–16.

10. Burgess, P. W., E. Veitcha, A. L. Costello, and T. Shallice. 1999. "The cognitive and neuroanatomical correlates of multitasking." *Neuropsychologia* 38(2000): 848–63.

11. Bloss, E. B., W. G. Janssen, B. S. McEwen and J. H. Morrison. 2010. "Interactive effects of stress and aging on structural plasticity in the prefrontal cortex." *Journal of Neuroscience* 30(19): 6726–31.

12. Vedhara, K., J. Hyde, I. D. Gilchrist, M. Tytherleigh, and S. Plummer. 2000. "Acute stress, memory, attention and cortisol." *Psychoneuroendocrinology* 25: 535–49.

13. McCormick, C. M., E. Lewis, B. Somley, and T. A. Kahan. 2007. "Individual differences in cortisol levels and performance on a test of executive function in men and women." *Physiology & Behavior* 91: 87–94.

14. Van der Linden, D., M. Frese and T. F. Meijman. 2003. "Mental fatigue and the control of cognitive processes: effects on perseveration and planning." *Acta Psychologica* 113: 45–65.

15. Levine, B., I. H. Robertson, L. Clare, G. Carter, J. Hong, B. A. Wilson, et al. 2000. "Rehabilitation of executive functioning: An experimental-clinical validation of goal management training." *Journal of the International Neuropsychological Society* 6(3): 299–312.

16. Just, M. A., T. A. Keller, and J. Cynkar. 2008. "A decrease in brain activation associated with driving when listening to someone speak." *Brain Research*. Author Manuscript: 1–22.

Chapter 5 Enhance Integrated Reasoning to Accelerate Performance

1. Chapman, S. B., S. Aslan, J. S. Spence, J. J. Hart, E. K. Bartz, N. Didehbani, et al. (2013). "Neural mechanisms of brain plasticity with complex cognitive training in healthy seniors." *Cerebral Cortex*. doi: 10.1093/cercor/bht234.

2. Fairlie, R. W. 2012. "2011 Kauffman index of entrepreneurial activity." *Ewing Marion Kauffman Foundation*: 1–32.

3. Duggan, T. 2007. *Strategic Intuition: The Creative Spark in Human Achievement*. Chichester, West Sussex, UK: Columbia University Press.

4. Anand, R., S. B. Chapman, A. Rackley, M. Keebler, J. Zientz, and J. Hart. 2011. "Gist reasoning training in cognitively normal seniors." *International Journal of Geriatric Psychiatry* 26 (9): 961–68.

5. Chapman et al. 2013. "Neural mechanisms of brain plasticity with complex cognitive training in healthy seniors." *Cerebral Cortex*. doi: 10.1093/cercor/bht234.

Chapter 6 Innovate to Inspire Your Thinking

1. Ward, T. B. 2004. "Cognition, creativity, and entrepreneurship." *Journal of Business Venturing* 19: 173–88.

2. Sternberg, R. J. 2006. "The Rainbow Project: Enhancing the SAT through assessments of analytical, practical, and creative skills." *Intelligence* 34(4): 321–50.

3. Leshner, A. 2011. "Innovation Needs Novel Thinking." *Science* 332(6033): 1009.

4. Goel, V. and R. J. Dolan. 2003. "Reciprocal neural response within lateral and ventral medial prefrontal cortex during hot and cold reasoning." *Neuro-Image* 20: 2314–21.

5. Draganskia, B. and A. May. 2008. "Training-induced structural changes in the adult human brain." *Behavioural Brain Research* 192: 137–42.

Section III Make Your Brain Smarter at Any Age
Chapter 7 The Immediates, 13–24 Years of Age

1. Jones, S., L. N. Clarke, S. Cornish, M. Gonzales, C. Johnson, J. N. Lawson, et al. 2002. "The Internet goes to college: How students are living in the future with today's technology." Pew Internet Project Survey, Pew Internet & American Life Project. http://www.pewinternet.org/~/media/Files/Reports/2002/PIP_College_Report.pdf.pdf.

2. Jones et al. "The Internet goes to college: How students are living in the future with today's technology."

3. Robinson, K. 2011. *Out of Our Minds: Learning to Be Creative.* Oxford, UK: Capstone Publishing Limited.

4. Zeldes, N., D. Sward, and S. Louchheim. 2007. "Infomania: Why we can't afford to ignore it any longer." *First Monday* 12(8–6).

5. Smith, C. 2011. *Lost in Transition: The Dark Side of Emerging Adulthood.* New York: Oxford University Press, Inc.

6. Ito, M. 2004. "'Nurturing the brain' as an emerging research field involving child neurology." *Brain & Development* 26: 429–33.

7. Bridgeland, J. M., J. J. Dilulio, Jr., and K. B. Morison. 2006. "The silent epidemic: perspectives of high school dropouts. A report by Civic Enterprises in association with Peter D. Hart Research Associates for the Bill & Melinda Gates Foundation."

8. Chapman, S. B., J. F. Gamino, and R. A. Mudar. 2012. "Higher order strategic gist reasoning in adolescence." In Reyna, V. F., S. B. Chapman, M. Dougherty, and J. Confrey (eds.), *The Adolescent Brain: Learning, Reasoning, and Decision Making.* Washington, DC: American Psychological Association.

9. Gogtay, N., J. N. Giedd, L. Lusk, K. M. Hayashi, D. Greenstein, A. C. Vaituzis, et al. 2004. "Dynamic mapping of human cortical development during childhood through early adulthood." Proceedings of the National Academy of Sciences of the United States of America 101(21): 8174–79.

10. Giedd, J. N., L. S. Clasen, R. Lenroot, D. Greenstein, G. L. Wallace, S. Ordaz, and G. P. Chrousos. 2006. "Puberty-related influences on brain development." *Mollecular and Cellular Endocrinology* 254–255: 154–62.

11. Gamino, J., S. B. Chapman, E. L. Hull, G. R. Lyon, G. R. 2010. "Effects of higher-order cognitive strategy training on gist reasoning and fact learning in adolescents." *Frontiers in Educational Psychology* 1.

12. Diamond, A. and K. Lee. 2011. "Interventions shown to aid executive function development in children 4 to 12 years old." *Science* 333(6045): 959–64.

13. Gamino et al. "Effects of higher-order cognitive strategy training on gist reasoning and fact learning in adolescents."

14. Perkins, R., G. Moran, J. Cosgrove, and G. Shield. 2010. "PISA 2009: The performance and progress of 15-year-olds in Ireland." Summary report. Dublin: Educational Research Centre.

15. Bridgeland et al. "The silent epidemic: perspectives of high school dropouts. A report by Civic Enterprises in association with Peter D. Hart Research Associates for the Bill & Melinda Gates Foundation."

16. Perkins et al. "PISA 2009: The performance and progress of 15-year-olds in Ireland."

17. Hanushek, E. A. and L. Woessmann. 2011. "How much do educational outcomes matter in OECD countries?" *Economic Policy* 26(67): 427–91.

Chapter 8 The Finders, 25–35, and the Seekers, 36–45 Years of Age

1. Sparrow, B., J. Liu, and D. M. Wegner. 2011. "Google effects on memory: cognitive consequences of having information at our fingertips." *Sciencexpress*, 1–6.

2. Bonahan, J. 2011. "Searching for the Google Effect on people's memory." Science 333(6040): 277.

3. Sparrow et al. "Google effects on memory: cognitive consequences of having information at our fingertips."

4. Lanier, J. 2010. "The end of human specialness." The Chronicle of Higher Education, 10th Anniversary Review. https://chronicle.com/article/The-End -of-Human-Specialness/124124/.

5. Carlile, P. R. 2004. "Transferring, translating, and transforming: An integrative framework for managing knowledge across boundaries." *Organization Science* 15(5): 555–68.

6. Lanier, J. 2010. *You Are Not a Gadget: A Manifesto*. New York: Alfred A. Knopf.

7. McCormick, C. M., E. Lewis, B. Somley, and T. A. Kahan. 2007. "Individual differences in cortisol levels and performance on a test of executive function in men and women." *Physiology & Behavior* 91: 87–94.

8. McEwen, B. S. 2007. "Physiology and neurobiology of stress and adaptation: Central role of the brain." *Physiological Review* 87: 873–904.

Chapter 9 The Thinkers, 46–65 Years of Age

1. MetLife Mature Market Institute. 2006. "Memory screening: Who attends and Why—A Survey of Participants at National Memory Screening Day." http://www.alzfdn.org/Surveys/survey1.pdf.

2. Salthouse, T. A. 2011. "Neuroanatomical substrates of age-related cognitive decline." *Psychological Bulletin* 137(5): 753–84.

3. Smith, C. 2011. *Lost in Transition: The Dark Side of Emerging Adulthood*. New York: Oxford University Press, Inc.

4. Valenzuela, M. J., M. Breakspear, and P. Sachdev. 2007. "Complex mental activity and the aging brain: Molecular, cellular and cortical network mechanisms." *Brain Research Reviews* 56(1): 198–213.

5. D'Esposito, M., and A. Gazzaley. 2011. "Can age-associated memory decline be treated?" *New England Journal Medicine* 365: 1346–47.

6. Rajah, M. N., S. Bastianetto, K. Bromley-Brits, R. Cools, M. D'Esposito, C. L. Grady, et al. 2009. "Biological changes associated with healthy versus pathological aging: A symposium review." *Ageing Research Reviews* 8(2): 140–146.

7. Salthouse. "Neuroanatomical substrates of age-related cognitive decline," 753–84.

8. Salthouse. "Neuroanatomical substrates of age-related cognitive decline," 753–84.

9. Preusse, F., E. Van der Meer, G. Deshpande, F. Krueger, and I. Wartenburger. 2011. "Fluid intelligence allows flexible recruitment of the parieto-frontal network in analogical reasoning." *Frontiers in Human Neuroscience* 5(22).

10. Greenwood, P. M. and R. Parasuraman. 2010. "Neuronal and cognitive plasticity: A neurocognitive framework for ameliorating cognitive aging." *Frontiers in Aging Neuroscience* 2: 150.

11. Valenzuela et al. "Complex mental activity and the aging brain: Molecular, cellular and cortical network mechanisms," 198–213.

12. Braver, T. S. 2012. "The variable nature of cognitive control: a dual mechanisms framework." *Trends in Cognitive Sciences* 16(2): 106–13.

13. Keeter, S. 2008. "The aging of the boomers and the rise of the millennials." In R. Teixeira (Ed.), *Red, Blue and Purple America: The Future of Election Demographics*. Washington, DC: Brookings Press: 225-57.

14. Bonahan, J. 2011. "Searching for the Google Effect on people's memory." *Science* 333(6040): 277.

15. Dumitriu, D., J. Hao, Y. Hara, J. Kaufmann, W. G. M. Janssen, W. Lou, et al. 2010. "Selective changes in thin spine density and morphology in monkey prefrontal cortex correlate with aging-related cognitive impairment." *Journal of Neuroscience* 30(22): 7507–15.

16. Salthouse. "Neuroanatomical substrates of age-related cognitive decline," 753–84.

17. MetLife Mature Market Institute. 2012. "Transitioning into retirement: the MetLife study of baby boomers at 65." http://www.metlife.com/assets/cao/mmi/publications/studies/2012/studies/mmi-transitioning-retirement.pdf.

18. Collins, J. 2001. *Good to Great: Why Some Companies Make the Leap . . . and Others Don't*. New York: HarperCollins.

19. "Boomers: The next 20 years." 2007. Institute for the Future. Pamphlet available at http://www.iftf.org.

Chapter 10 The Knowers, 66–100+ Years of Age

1. Delbanco, N. 2011. *Lastingness: The art of old age*. New York: Grand Central Publishing.

2. Dana, R. 2012. "'Nevertirees': Elderly Americans who refuse to retire." *Newsweek*. Retrieved from http://www.thedailybeast.com/newsweek/2012/03/11/nevertirees-elderly-americans-who-refuse-to-retire.html.

3. Friedman, H. S. and L. R. Martin. 2011. *The Longevity Project: Surprising Discoveries for Health and Long Life from the Landmark Eight-Decade Study*. New York: Hudson Street Press.

4. Grossmann, I., J. Na, M. E. W. Varnum, D. C. Park, S. Kitayama and R. E. Nisbett. 2010. "Reasoning about social conflicts improves into old age." *Proceedings of the National Academy of Sciences of the United States of America* 107(16): 7246–50.

5. Coombes, A. 2007. "Happy days ahead." *The Wall Street Journal: Market Watch*. http://articles.marketwatch.com/2007-08-05/finance/30812757_1_younger-people-happy-days-laura-carstensen.

6. Lancaster, L. C. and D. Stillman. 2002. *When Generations Collide: Who They Are. Why They Clash. How to Solve the Generational Puzzle at Work*. New York: HarperCollins.

7. Kane, S. 2012. "The true recipe for workplace complexity." *BusinessDay Online*. http://businessdayonline.com/NG/index.php/work/33088-the-true-recipe-for-workplace-complexity.

8. Berns, G. S., D. Laibson, and G. Loewenstein. 2007. "Intertemporal choice—toward an integrative framework." *Trends in Cognitive Sciences* 11(11): 482–88.

9. Wilson, R. S., E. Segawa, P. A. Boyle, and D. A. Bennett. 2012. "Influence of late-life cognitive activity on cognitive health." *Neurology* 78(15): 1123–29.

10. Rohwedder, S. and R. J. Willis. 2010. "Mental Retirement." *Journal of Economic Perspectives* 24(1): 119–38.

11. Oz, M. 2011. "Why work is good for brain health: Studies show staying active is good for your body and mind." *AARP The Magazine* May/June 2011.

12. Vedhara K., J. Hyde, I. D. Gilchrist, M. Tytherleigh, and S. Plummer. 2000. "Acute stress, memory, attention and cortisol." *Psychoneuroendocrinology* 25: 535–49.

13. Chrousos, G. P. 2009. "Stress and disorders of the stress system." *National Review Endocrinology* 5: 374–81.

14. Bennis, W. and P. W. Biederman. 2010. *Still Surprised: A Memoir of a Life in Leadership*. New York: Jossey-Bass.

15. Anand, R., S. B. Chapman, A. Rackley, M. Keebler, J. Zientz, and J. Hart. 2011. "Gist reasoning training in cognitively normal seniors." *International Journal of Geriatric Psychiatry* 26(9): 961–68.

16. Chapman, S. B., J. Zientz, M. Weiner, R. Rosenberg, W. Frawley, and M. H. Burns. 2002. "Discourse changes in early Alzheimer disease, mild cognitive impairment, and normal aging." *Alzheimer Disease and Associated Disorders* 16(3): 177–86.

17. Ulatowska, H. K., S. B. Chapman, A. P. Highly, and J. Prince. 1998. "Discourse in healthy old-elderly adults: A longitudinal study." *Aphasiology* 12(7/8): 619–33.

18. Fairlie, R. W. 2012. "2011 Kauffman index of entrepreneurial activity." Ewing Marion Kauffman Foundation: 1–32.

19. Foubert-Samier, A., G. Catheline, H. Amieva, B. Dilharreguy, C. Helmer, M. Allard, and J. F. Dartigues, 2010. "Education, occupation, leisure activities, and brain reserve: a population-based study." *Neurobiology of Aging* 33(2): 423.e15.

20. Anand et al. "Gist reasoning training in cognitively normal seniors," 961–68.

21. Chapman, S. B., C. W. Cotman, H. M. Fillit, M. Gallagher, and C. H. van Dyck. 2012. "Clinical trials: New opportunities." *Journals of Gerontology Series A: Biological Sciences and Medical Sciences*: 1–13.

22. Chapman, S. B., S. Aslan, J. S. Spence, J. J. Hart, E. K. Bartz, N. Didehbani, et al. (2013). "Neural mechanisms of brain plasticity with complex cognitive training in healthy seniors." *Cerebral Cortex*. doi: 10.1093/cercor/bht234.

Section IV Mind the Gap in Injury and Disease
Chapter 11 Rebound and Rewire Your Brain After Injury

1. Rao, V. and C. Lyketsos. 2000. "Neuropsychiatric sequelae of traumatic brain Injury." *Psychosomatics* 41(2): 95–103.
2. Rehabilitation of persons with Traumatic Brain Injury. NIH Consensus Statement Online 1998 Oct 26-2816(1): 1–41.
3. Marquez de la Plata, C., F. G. Yang, J. Y. Wang, K. Krishnan, K. Bakhadirov, C. Paliotta, et al. 2011. "Diffusion tensor imaging biomarkers for traumatic axonal injury: Analysis of three analytic methods." *Journal of the International Neuropsychological Society* 17: 24–35.
4. Guskiewicz, K. M., S. W. Marshall, J. Bailes, M. McCrea, H. P. Harding, Jr., A. Matthews, et al. 2007. "Recurrent concussion and risk of depression in retired professional football players." *Medicine and Science in Sports & Exercise* 39(6): 903–9.
5. Chen, A. J. W., G. M. Abrams, and M. D'Esposito, M. 2006. "Functional reintegration of prefrontal neural networks for enhancing recovery after brain injury." *Journal of Head Trauma Rehabilitation* 21(2): 107.
6. Max, W., E. J. MacKenzie, and D. P. Rice. 1991. "Head injuries: Cost and consequences." *Journal of Head Trauma Rehabilitation* 6: 76–91.
7. Benson, R. R., S. A. Meda, S. Vasudevan, Z. Kou, K. A. Govindarajan, R. A. Hanks, et al. 2007. "Global white matter analysis of diffusion tensor images is predictive of injury severity in traumatic brain injury." *Journal of Neurotrauma* 3: 446–59.
8. Benson et al. "Global white matter analysis of diffusion tensor images is predictive of injury severity in traumatic brain injury," 446–59.
9. Vas, A. K., S. B. Chapman, L. G. Cook, A. C. Elliott, and M. Keebler. 2011. "Higher-order reasoning training years after traumatic brain injury in adults." *The Journal of Head Trauma Rehabilitation* 26(3): 224–39.
10. Vas, A., S. B. Chapman, D. Krawczyk, K. Krishnan, and M. Keebler. 2010. "Executive control training to enhance frontal plasticity in traumatic brain injury." International Brain Injury Association's Eighth World Congress on Brain Injury, *Brain Injury* 24(3): 115–463.
11. Chen et al. "Functional reintegration of prefrontal neural networks for enhancing recovery after brain injury," 107.

12. Benson et al. "Global white matter analysis of diffusion tensor images is predictive of injury severity in traumatic brain injury," 446–59.

13. Cook, L. G., R. DePompei, and S. B. Chapman. 2010. "Cognitive communicative challenges in TBI: Assessment and intervention in the long term." *ASHA Perspectives, Division 2.*

14. Vas, Chapman, Cook, et al. "Higher-order reasoning training years after traumatic brain injury in adults," 224–39.

15. McCauley, S. R., C. Pedroza, S. B. Chapman, L. G. Cook, A. C. Vásquez, and H. S. Levin. 2011. "Monetary incentive effects on event-based prospective memory three months after traumatic brain injury in children." *Journal of Clinical and Experimental Neuropsychology* 33(6): 639–46.

16. McCauley et al. "Monetary incentive effects on event-based prospective memory three months after traumatic brain injury in children," 639–46.

17. Chen et al. "Functional reintegration of prefrontal neural networks for enhancing recovery after brain injury," 107.

18. Lomber, S. G., M. A. Meredith and A. Kral. 2010. "Cross-modal plasticity in specific auditory cortices underlies visual compensations in the deaf." *Nature Neuroscience* 13(11): 1421–29.

19. Vas, Chapman, Cook, et al. "Higher-order reasoning training years after traumatic brain injury in adults," 224–39.

20. Max et al. "Head injuries: Cost and consequences," 76–91.

21. National Center for Injury Prevention and Control. 2003. "Report to Congress on Mild Traumatic Brain Injury in the United States: Steps to Prevent a Serious Public Health Problem." Atlanta, GA: Centers for Disease Control and Prevention.

Chapter 12 Stave Off Decline in Alzheimer's

1. Chapman, S. B., J. Zientz, M. Weiner, R. Rosenberg, W. Frawley, and M. H. Burns. 2002. "Discourse changes in early Alzheimer disease, mild cognitive impairment, and normal aging." *Alzheimer Disease and Associated Disorders* 16(3): 177–86.

2. Chapman, S. B., J. F. Gamino, L. G. Cook, G. Hanten, X. Li, and H. S. Levin. 2006. "Impaired discourse gist and working memory in children after brain injury." *Brain and Language* 97: 178–88.

3. Chapman, S. B. and H. K. Ulatowska. 1997. "Discourse in dementia: Consideration of consciousness." In M. I. Stamenov (Ed.), *Language Structure, Discourse and the Access to Consciousness.* Philadelphia: John Benjamin Publishing Company: 155–88.

4. Alzheimer's Association. http://www.alz.org/research/science/alzheimers_re search.asp.

5. Alzheimer's Association. "What is the economic impact of Alzheimer's disease?" http://alzheimers.factsforhealth.org/what/impact.asp.

6. Acevedo, A. and D. A. Loewenstein. 2007. "Nonpharmacological cognitive interventions in aging and dementia." *Journal of Geriatric Psychiatry and Neurology* 20(4): 239–49.

7. Eisler, R. and D. S. Levine. 2002. "Nurture, nature, and caring: We are not prisoners of our genes." *Brain and Mind* 3: 9–52.

8. Erickson, K. I., R. S. Prakash, M. W. Voss, L. Chaddock, L. Hu, K. S. Morris, et al. (2009). "Aerobic fitness is associated with hippocampal volume in elderly humans." *Hippocampus* 19(10), 1030–39.

9. Chapman, Zientz, et al. "Discourse changes in early Alzheimer disease, mild cognitive impairment, and normal aging," 177–86.

10. Rackley, A. and S. Dembling. 2009. *I Can Still Laugh: Stories of Inspiration and Hope from Individuals Living with Alzheimer's.* Charleston, SC: BookSurge Publishing.

11. Chapman, S. B., C. W. Cotman, H. M. Fillit, M. Gallagher, and C. H. van Dyck. 2012. "Clinical trials: New opportunities." *Journals of Gerontology Series A: Biological Sciences and Medical Sciences*: 1–13.

12. Erickson et al. "Aerobic fitness is associated with hippocampal volume in elderly humans," 1030–39.

13. Ruscheweyh, R., C. Willemer, K. Kruger, T. Duning, T. Warnecke, J. Sommer, et al. 2011. "Physical activity and memory functions: An interventional study." *Neurobiology of Aging* 32(7), 1304–19.

INDEX

ABOUT THE AUTHORS

Sandra Bond Chapman, Ph.D., founder and chief director of the Center for BrainHealth, is a Distinguished Professor at The University of Texas at Dallas in the School of Behavioral and Brain Sciences. Known for thirty years of innovative discovery, she is recognized as a leading thinker in transforming how people, young and old, can build a smarter brain. A cognitive neuroscientist with more than forty fully funded research grants, Dr. Chapman collaborates with scientists across the country and around the world to solve some of the most important issues concerning the brain and its health. Dr. Chapman's scientific study elucidates these issues and applies novel approaches to advance creative and critical thinking, to strengthen healthy brain development, and to incite innovation throughout life. She lives in Dallas with her husband, Don.

Shelly Kirkland, public relations director at the Center for BrainHealth at The University of Texas at Dallas, brings national attention to the cutting-edge research facility dedicated to understanding, protecting, and healing the brain. She lives in Dallas with her husband, Keith.